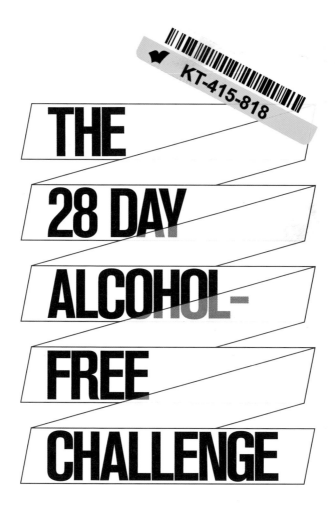

THE

28 DAY

ALCOHOL-

FREE

CHALLENGE

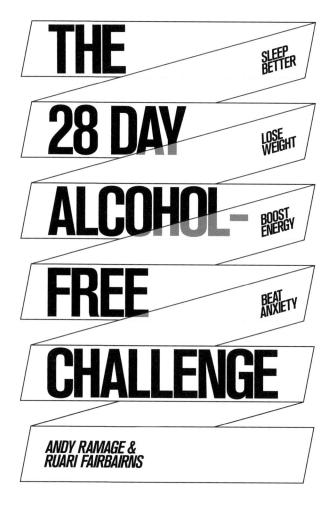

THE
28 DAY
ALCOHOL-
FREE
CHALLENGE

SLEEP BETTER

LOSE WEIGHT

BOOST ENERGY

BEAT ANXIETY

**ANDY RAMAGE &
RUARI FAIRBAIRNS**

bluebird
books for life

First published 2017 by Bluebird
an imprint of Pan Macmillan
20 New Wharf Road, London N1 9RR
Associated companies throughout the world
www.panmacmillan.com

ISBN 978-1-5098-5725-8

3 5 7 9 8 6 4

A CIP catalogue record for this book is available from
the British Library.

Printed in Italy

Visit www.panmacmillan.com to read more about all our books and to buy
them. You will also find features, author interviews and news of any author
events, and you can sign up for e-newsletters so that you're always first to hear
about our new releases.

DEDICATIONS

To my wife Jen, thank you for being my rock. For listening to me bang on forever and still love me, for trusting me enough to lay down your soul and grow with me. To my beautiful girls, Tillie and Robin, for being my reason why. To my parents for creating this ball of energy, and to my siblings and family, for helping to shape that energy into what it is today.
– *Ruari*

I would like to thank my amazing, wondrous wife for her never-ending support and for editing every single word I write. Her unconditional love has allowed me to take on these madcap adventures and have a great time in the process. I would also like to thank my girls Molly and Ruby who inspire me every single day. Finally I have to say thank you to my parents Kath and Jim for giving me the best start in life anyone could ask for.
–*Andy*

CONTENTS

In 2015, Professor Kevin Moore of the Royal Free Hospital, in London, co-authored one of the largest ever studies into the effects of a four-week break from alcohol. The participants were average drinkers who were taking part in the Dry January campaign and the results were staggering.

By the end of the four weeks, the participants of the studies had each lost, on average, 40 per cent of their liver fat and 3kg in weight, and also had reduced cholesterol and lower glucose levels.

Moore was so impressed with the findings that he suggested that if there were a pill that produced similar results, everyone would want it.

This book is that pill.

OUR STORY

It's hard to fathom that we are here writing a book to help you experience a period of life alcohol-free when only a few years ago we were the party boys, the larger-than-life characters, first-in-last-out-of-the-bar type lads, knee deep in booze. So let's set the record straight from the off: we had some good times over our drinking careers and we are certainly not here to judge. If you're still loving life and achieving everything you want while drinking, that's great for you. But if, like us, you have reached a point where you suspect alcohol is holding you back, join us on this inspirational adventure and we will show you exactly how to regain total control of your body and life.

Perhaps you've been motivated to do a month-long alcohol-free challenge for charity, or maybe you just want to quietly take a break to prove that you can. Whatever your reasons, you've made a great first step by picking up this book.

A tipping point is on the horizon, with the world waking up to the fact that life is so much brighter without booze. Millennials are drinking less, 'sober curious' is becoming hip, and the peak levels of alcohol consumption in the UK were reached back in 2004[1]. The cool kids are now alcohol-free. Entrepreneurs, film stars and sporting heroes are all coming to the same conclusion: there is no place for hangovers and lethargy in their best and most-accomplished lives.

As luck would have it, we both stumbled upon the realisation that alcohol was preventing us being our best at a similar moment. Suddenly hangovers were hanging around for days. We felt tired and lethargic most of the time. The sparkle of daily life was fading into a merry-go-round of nights out and surviving, rather than loving life.

To be clear, there was no rock bottom, epiphany or doctor's note. We just wanted to be better dads, better professionals, healthier, fitter, faster, leaner, and we suspected our drinking habits were holding us back. But to even question the alcohol situation sent shivers down our spines. Our worlds had been built around alcohol. It was how we socialised and how we met new clients and built our business. Our friendships were formed over beer and our wives both enjoyed a drink. Yet we couldn't shake the feeling that this pastime was somehow preventing us getting the most out of life – even though social pressure was yelling the opposite. We both knew that the only way to uncover the truth was to take a decent break.

So we set ourselves a challenge: one year, no beer. But before we could entertain the thought of 365 days alcohol-free, our mission was to get through the first month.

It was during these first 28 days that we got a taster of how much brighter our lives could be. This experience gave us the courage to continue, and for this reason we both feel that this 28-day challenge is the perfect place to start. You will get a glimpse of how life will be without alcohol, and whether you decide to continue at the end of the challenge or not, your relationship with alcohol will already have begun to change.

Doubts emerged very quickly. Would we still be funny? Would our mates desert us? Would our wives think us boring? Then there were the direct threats from people we admired, who had already hinted that our blossoming careers would be over if we did not entertain clients over drinks. But we didn't care; we were on a mission to experience all that an alcohol-free life had to offer and to see if booze was holding us back. We both came to the same conclusion pretty quickly: it was.

After a few false starts, trips, slips and departures from the wagon, we were off on our alcohol-free mission. That was when things got exciting. Rather than our lives falling apart as we feared, they improved beyond compare. It transpires that quitting alcohol opened the door to the lives we had always wanted. The energy, motivation and vitality that came flooding back to us took our productivity to new levels.

As the fog of hangovers lifted, we noticed which types of food nourished our bodies and minds. From this vantage point we adjusted our diets accordingly. This gave us more energy, which helped us to make the gym sessions that we used to avoid. In turn, regular exercise helped improve our mental fitness, which reduced stress and provided extra vitality to train. We had kick-started an upward spiral as each improvement led to further improvements.

Slowly but surely we smashed the conventional wisdom and social pressure that insisted we needed alcohol to have fun and to live a full life. In fact, we discovered at first hand that the opposite was true. On a personal and business level, our relationships blossomed, putting to rest one of our biggest fears. We also found that we had so much more time, revealing that drinking – and the resulting hangovers – had been stealing precious moments from our days. As the quality of our sleep improved, we both experimented with 5 a.m. starts. We couldn't believe it; rather than giving something up, we found that we gained by uncovering a wealth of new and inspiring advantages.

As our appreciation of these advantages deepened, our frustration with the conventional wisdom around drinking grew. We realised there must be millions of people just like us who are overwhelmed by the combination of this 'wisdom' and social pressure. We knew that if these people had the chance to experience life alcohol-free for long enough, they would probably change their relationship with alcohol forever, and in doing so change their lives.

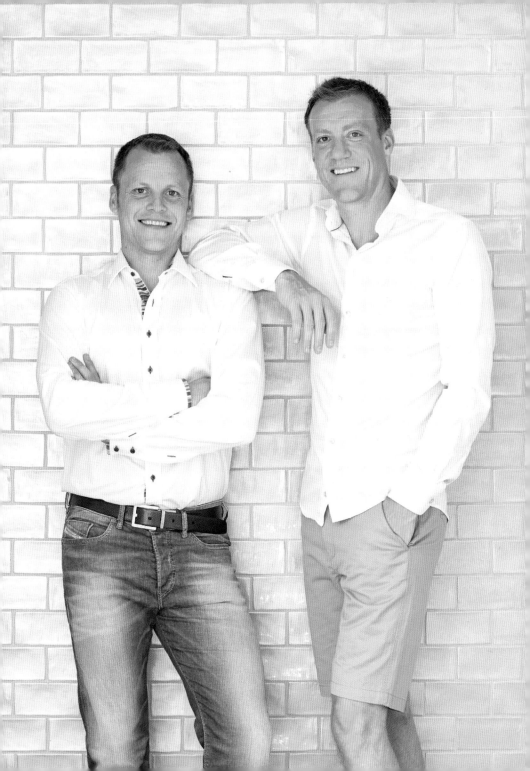

A FRESH APPROACH

**Having searched both online and offline groups within the alcohol-free
space, we struggled to find a collective that shared our ethos.
Although many of these groups were helping lots of people, they held
zero appeal for us. The vast majority were based around the belief
that alcohol is something you have to give up and will always want,
but we believe that a very different, more positive approach can lead to
a healthier relationship with booze. Also, lots of these groups fostered
a negative approach to habit-change. After reading a few comments on
their forums we felt down and defeated, which was the polar opposite
to the mindset we were thinking of. We didn't want to bang on about
the negatives, we wanted to sing from the rooftops about all the good
things that can happen when you take a break from booze.**

So when we couldn't find a tribe that
supported our goals, we thought, why
not create our own? In that moment
OneYearNoBeer (OYNB) was born.

This was our mission:

*'To help as many people as possible change their
relationship with alcohol completely.'*

This could mean that someone who
has reached the end of their alcohol-free
challenge might choose to drink every now
and then in full control, or they might
continue with their challenge or possibly
even never drink again. The choice is theirs.
Our objective was to help people regain
control of their drinking habits, whatever
form that might take.

So we started by creating a website and a
Facebook group. At this early stage we both
agreed that if our stories and this community
could help just one or two people it would
be a success. We had absolutely no idea that
what was about to happen would change the
course of our lives.

Within a few weeks we had tens of
thousands of people from over 671 cities and
71 different countries signing up to the
website and taking the 90-day alcohol-free
challenge. This blew our minds – and it still
does today. We both feel so proud to be part
of an amazing group that continues to support
and inspire each other on a daily basis.
OneYearNoBeer would be nothing without
these amazing individuals who have come
together to create something truly special.

As the tribe started to grow, so did our drive to inspire more people. We wanted the world to know that going alcohol-free was advantageous, not a sacrifice. So we created blogs, podcasts and webinars to help spread the word. At the same time, physical meet-ups started across the world, from Vancouver to Dublin. Role models were coming forward to make a stand and inspire us that you can live a fantastic life alcohol-free. The power of the tribe was working – on an epic scale.

Our next objective was to combine the power of this alcohol-free tribe with a world-class habit-change model. So we studied the psychology of change and created a unique mental and physical system – MEND – to support our OYNBers on their alcohol-free adventures.

The MEND system (see page 38), which we use for this 28-day challenge, was informed by our own experience of the challenge and that of our members, which was combined with the best bits from positive psychology, behavioural science, science of habit-change, NLP (Neuro-Linguistic Programming), mindfulness, physical exercise and nutrition. We are not so much standing on the shoulders of giants, but pirouetting on their rather bright heads.

To be clear, we do not have all the answers when it comes to habit-change, and there is a constant and neverending quest for improvement. But having now helped thousands of people change their relationship with alcohol, we feel that all the hard work is starting to pay off.

OUR OBJECTIVE IS TO HELP PEOPLE REGAIN CONTROL, IN WHATEVER FORM THAT TAKES.

NOTE
If you feel that you are in any way dependent on alcohol, please seek a doctor's advice before starting this challenge.

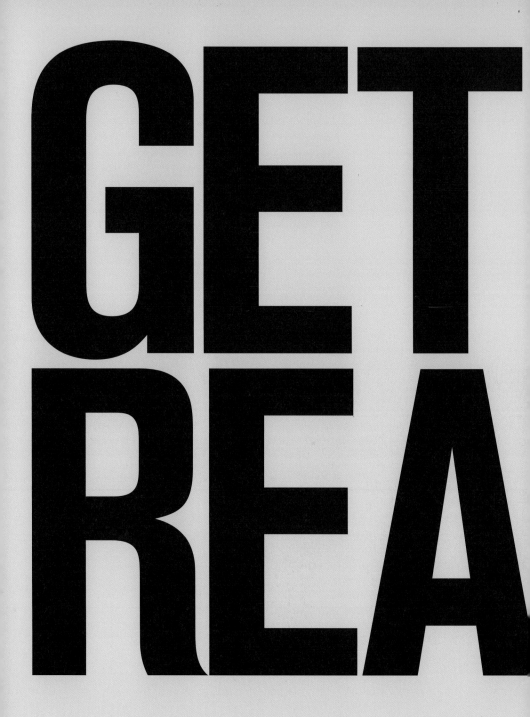

THE 28-DAY CHAMPION CHALLENGE

We both love a challenge – from learning new skills to running marathons – and so did our friends, it seemed; it felt as though every week someone we knew was taking some sort of challenge. So we thought, why not try an alcohol-free one? Most would agree that this is a mighty social challenge and one that's worth total respect.

When we set up OYNB we created two challenges: the 90-day hero and the 365-day legend. But we also wanted to create a shorter version which would allow even more people to enjoy a break from booze. With Dry January and Sober October becoming more and more popular, we wanted a challenge that would inspire people for a month, at any time of year.

So we decided to take all the best bits from our 90- and 365-day challenges and condense them into a 28-day champion challenge, just for you. This way you get to experience all the great tips, tricks and hacks over the course of four weeks. Also, 28 days feels much more achievable when compared to a year. But what we know is this: if you can do 28 days, you can do 90 days, and if you can do 90, you can do the year. So think

of this 28-day champion challenge as a taster. Then at the end of this challenge you can decide whether your break is over and you return to normal, drink every now and then in full control, continue with the challenge or never drink again. The choice is yours.

What's great about this 28-day challenge is that in this short space of time the research suggests that you might lose weight, lower cholesterol, improve blood pressure, reduce your risk of diabetes and sleep better. Also you will start to experience all those other alcohol-free benefits, such as more time, energy and motivation, an improved social life and the confidence that you can create a vibrant, healthy lifestyle without booze.

So let's get ready. But before we do – a warning: from now on your relationship with alcohol will change forever.

KICK-START YOUR CHALLENGE ONLINE

Before starting this week we highly recommend you join our online OneYearNoBeer community: oneyearnobeer. com. The private forums and Facebook groups will provide extra support and inspiration.

You can also sign up to one of our online alcohol-free challenge packages which provide daily email support, daily video support, exclusive webinars, audio support and one of the most amazing

communities on the net. Finally, if you use the exclusive promo code '28daybook' at sign up we will refund you the price of this book!

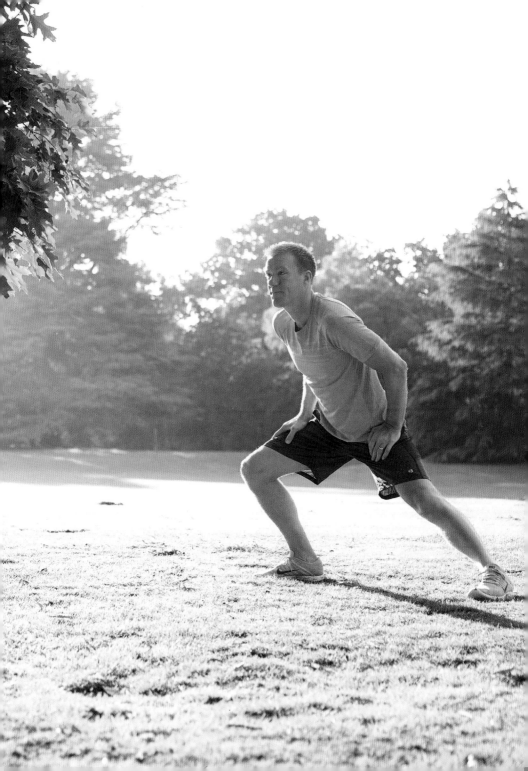

SLEEP LIKE A BABY

Sleep is absolutely key to a healthy lifestyle, yet it is often completely underrated. Let's not beat around the proverbial bush – alcohol has the ability to destroy sleep. Late nights deprive you of precious hours, but the real damage is caused by poor-quality sleep. Even a small amount of alcohol has been shown to break sleep patterns by not allowing you to reach deep healing sleep, so your body cannot recover sufficiently[2]. You wake feeling tired, lethargic and often anxious. Many people then compound this problem by using alcohol to send them off to the sandman, but they fail to recognise that the quality of this sleep is so poor they are left constantly tired. It's a false economy.

> *I am sleeping like a log! Waking up at 6 a.m. and getting shit done. I love this. This is the longest stretch I have had with no alcohol in around 25 years!*
>
> *CHRIS*

Studies suggest that if you don't get enough sleep, you might:

— **Struggle with concentration**
— **Become accident-prone**
— **Lack willpower**
— **Become less productive**
— **Increase your risk of a heart attack**
— **Raise the risk of becoming overweight**
— **If that's not enough – you also increase your risk of dying early!**

One of life's best feelings is waking up after a great night's sleep, full of vitality and ready to take on the world. Quality sleep is the engine that powers a healthy, vibrant lifestyle. After a few weeks alcohol-free we both started to notice the difference. As the nagging tiredness lifted, our motivation and productivity increased, which in turn fed so many of the alcohol-free advantages. Quality sleep was another massive bonus that we totally overlooked when we first considered taking a break.

Finally, many of our members who used alcohol as a sleeping pill found sleeping tricky at first, but those who persevered reported life-changing benefits from the improved quality of their sleep.

THE GATEWAY TO BETTER HEALTH

The health benefits from going alcohol-free far exceed the obvious – as you are about to discover.

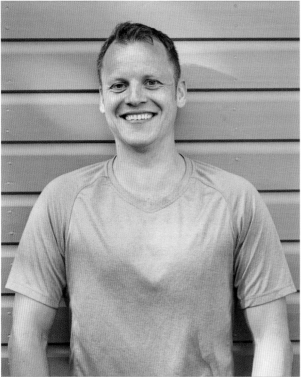

Do you want to lose weight easily, lose belly bloat, have clearer skin, reduce wrinkles and fine lines, get better sleep, improve digestion, eliminate brain fog, think more clearly, be more productive, have more energy, reduce anxiety, have more time for exercise, be able to choose healthier foods, and generally just feel fantastic? Are you ready? In fact, you'll even save yourself an enormous amount of money! So what could this miracle be? NOT drinking alcohol is the magic bullet you've all been searching for!

CHRISSIE

RUARI'S STORY

When drinking I felt constantly tired and would often end up having a few on social occasions to try to wake myself up. This was another vicious circle – alcohol ruined my sleep, which made me tired and lethargic, which I then attempted to overcome by drinking. Guess what? The next day I felt tired and lethargic and ordered another drink to get over it.

THE TRIPLE WHAMMY

What most books fail to mention about alcohol are the knock-on effects. Waking up with a hangover is not the end of the problem. When we really started to analyse what was happening in our worlds we noticed that the follow-on effects were doing twice as much damage. We were constantly hit with the triple whammy of:

— **Zero interest in exercise**
— **Craving rubbish food**
— **Emotional anxiety.**

This triple whammy plagued us for days after a drinking session. Very often we dropped exercise routines in favour of junk food and that anxious, just-not-right feeling hung around long afterwards.

Going alcohol-free was a turning point in our overall health. At the start of our challenge we considered ourselves pretty healthy guys. We were alive, which was a good place to start. Although slightly overweight, we were still pretty active. Our 1–2 spin classes each month and the odd 5k run were proof that we still had it. There were no obvious diseases to speak of, blood pressure was all good, cholesterol a little high but, all in all, we thought we were doing ok. Neither of us was initially motivated to stop drinking for any obvious health reasons.

We just assumed we were healthy because we weren't sick. However, a key lesson that we learnt over the following years is that the absence of illness does not imply health.

Just because right now, in this moment, you're not sick, it does not mean you're healthy. Too many of us are living stressful lives, eating poor diets, drinking too much, rarely exercising and making the assumption that we're ok – because currently, we are ok. The problem with this approach is that one day you will not be ok. You will be sick because of the way you lived while you weren't sick.

RUARI'S STORY

I had this mantra in my head that my willpower was poor. Therefore committing to trying to reduce certain foods always started well, but ended shortly after. That was until I went alcohol-free. Suddenly people around me were telling me I had incredible willpower, so I tried a Paleo diet with the faith that I would complete the diet for 90 days. If I could do booze, I could do anything. The diet changes had further dramatic effects on me; I established that I wasn't a long-time sufferer of IBS, I was lactose intolerant! It took the fog of alcohol and the mist of demotivation to dissipate to see the truth.

We were both a little guilty of this mindset. In truth, we never really stopped long enough to look at our overall health. We were too busy working hard to make our way in the world and to provide for our families. Then we stopped drinking and everything changed.

A GREAT TIME TO CLEAN UP YOUR DIET

Once we removed alcohol from our lives, we instantly dropped calories. One large strong beer is the caloric equivalent of a hot dog and fries. Imagine eating 10 of those on a night out! We do appreciate that alcohol is often swapped for other high-calorie drinks, so it was not just alcohol-free savings that were making the difference for us. The real game changer was that we no longer craved the late-night kebab and day-after pizza. This is where the big gains were made.

Another bonus of this alcohol-free lifestyle was that we started to notice how certain foods affected our mood and body. No longer could we blame the afternoon slump on last night's drinking session – we realised it had to be connected to the food we ate. For example, high-sugar foods caused our blood sugar to soar, then when it came crashing down, so did our energy. This is not rocket science – you are what you eat. Quitting alcohol created the space to review everything about our worlds. For this reason, so many of our OYNB members lose weight and get into the very best shape of their lives.

ANDY'S STORY

The combination of quality nutrition and exercise helped me lose a lot of weight. After only a few months I had lost 3 stone (42 lbs) and my body fat dropped from 30 per cent down to below 10 per cent, where it remains today. My cholesterol dropped from 3.0 to 1.2 and – most amazing of all – my resting heart rate plummeted from 64 to 48. At age 42, I was in better health than I had been when I was playing professional sport.

ALCOHOL HAS A LOT OF CALORIES … YOU MIGHT BE ALARMED TO SEE HOW MANY!

1 pint of 4% ABV (alcohol by volume) beer = 182 calories. Equivalent to one average chocolate bar.

330ml bottle of 5% ABV beer = 142 calories. Equivalent to a 25g bag of crisps.

1 pint of 4.5% ABV cider = 216 calories. Equivalent to three chipolata sausages.

175ml glass of 13% ABV wine = 159 calories. Equivalent to a slice of toast with a thin spread of butter.

MOTIVATION TO EXERCISE

As we've mentioned, ask any personal trainer and they will tell you that the number one reason why people cancel training sessions is because of a hangover. It's sad but true – and we had both been there.

As our alcohol-free vitality soared, so did our motivation to get fit. This was a massive gain for us both. Suddenly exercise was back on the cards in a big way. This presented a real opportunity to get a decent streak of exercising under our belts without it being ruined by a stray night on the sauce – much to the delight of our gym instructors.

Another key point is that exercise is not all about the obvious gym session. With hangovers out of the way and energy in abundance, we built stealth exercise into our lives. We started walking and sometimes even running to work. We also used the stairs instead of the lift. By treating our lives like a sports field we were discovering opportunities to create exercise as we went about our daily routines.

So whether you're a Sunday morning footballer, Pilates wannabe, yoga bunny, aspiring marathon runner, badminton fiend, netball fanatic, or just want to give your dog more exercise, quitting alcohol will make an enormous difference to your abilities.

MENTAL WELL-BEING SKYROCKETS

We don't want to bang on about all the terrible effects alcohol has on physical health. We all know that excessive drinking can lead to higher risks of cancer, depression, diabetes, hypertension, brain damage and dementia.

The key is doing something about it, and this is what we are here to help you achieve.

Of course, quitting alcohol is not a panacea for those suffering from serious mental health challenges such as anxiety and depression, for example, but it does provide a massive boost to those who suffer debilitating feelings after a drinking session. With a clear head from zero alcohol the world looks brighter and your emotional well-being is spared any alcohol-induced battering on the morning after the night before. This helps create an upward spiral of well-being.

When we started out on this challenge we had no idea just how much our

> *It's incredible to see the difference two months in to my OYNB challenge. I woke up at the age of 42 with a spare tyre around my middle, high cholesterol, a bloated face and just thought 'what am I doing to myself?'. Eight weeks in and I have lost three inches around my waist, six pounds in weight, my cholesterol has gone from 6.5 to 4.5, my skin feels ten years younger and my fitness level just gets better and better. I feel amazing and like I've had a complete body MOT.*
>
> **ELAINE**

mental and physical health would improve. This was another great example of the hidden benefits that only surfaced once we were alcohol-free.

BETTER RELATIONSHIPS

When most people first consider taking a break from booze, they imagine the future and worry about their relationships. This is a natural concern, and one that we felt intensely, too. We worried that we would no longer be considered one of the lads and genuinely feared that our business would decline. These are powerful concerns and ones that are echoed by thousands of our members.

For others, it might be the way a couple connect, relaxing after a long day with a glass of wine, or perhaps just how you always meet friends – in bars, clubs or restaurants over a drink.

We were both so scared of this particular problem that we were fully prepared to abandon the challenge if our business relationships slipped in the slightest.

Luckily, going alcohol-free allowed us to address these fears in the real world and to discover, quite early on, that our relationships were not struggling, but blossoming.

FAMILY

One of the biggest advantages our members notice is an improvement in personal relationships. This runs in total contrast to the conventional wisdom that social relationships are built upon and revolve around alcohol. Our newfound energy, vitality and clarity of mind allowed us to be truly present with our loved ones. In addition, having the time and motivation to contribute to home life made a massive difference to our families. The kids loved having dads who were on the ball and up for playing, messing around and generally having fun, instead of being grumpy and easily angered. This drove home the point that life is too short and children grow up too quickly for us to miss out on them because of a self-inflicted illness. Wasting a precious weekend nursing a hangover was simply no longer an option.

FRIENDS

We feared that friendships would fall apart without the alcohol glue, but once again the opposite was true. It's surprising how many mates were looking for an excuse to have a night off or do something different. It was not long before our friends went out of their way to organise social events that did not involve alcohol, to support our new healthy lifestyles. This led to more experiences, laughs and special moments that are worth so much more than a few drinks.

On the flip side, as our friendships evolved we found ourselves seeing less of some people and more of others. The reality is that some friendships won't be the same, but our alcohol-free adventure gifted us the chance to discover where our true friendships were. This allowed us to nurture and improve on the important relationships in our lives.

Finally, we both feel privileged that the OYNB community has opened us up to many more powerful friendships with likeminded and inspirational people.

WORK

This was a biggie. Could we still form lasting relationships without the business lubricant of alcohol? The answer was an emphatic yes. We found this fascinating because we were told in no uncertain terms that going alcohol-free would harm our careers. Admittedly, we had to adapt. While we still had the option of a drinks night, we wanted to play to our strengths, so we started to try new things. Who would have thought that

I'm happier and I have much more faith in myself. I'm hopeful for a wonderful future and for the first time I truly believe I can now see what I'm capable of. And my marriage has improved ten-fold! I'm much nicer, much more focused towards my wife and family, which makes my wife happier. I see a future as a fit and thoughtful husband and father who is prepared to enjoy his life to the fullest.

MICHAEL

clients and mates would get such a buzz from spin classes, surf trips and Barry's boot camp? Best of all, they really appreciated the extra effort we made to find unique and interesting activities to do with them.

Admittedly, we now spend less time in the bar with the lads, so there is a small argument that these relationships could be deeper. But when compared to all the other positives, this is a small price to pay. Also, life has a funny way of helping you gravitate towards those people who share your values. By going alcohol-free, there is a chance to make new and more interesting relationships.

MINE IS A SINGLE

Initially many of our single members worry about going on dates and meeting new people without alcohol. We totally get this – it feels as though most social occasions that might offer the chance to meet someone special are fuelled by booze. But our single members are discovering that there are many benefits to retaining a clear head when you are out socially:

— It's a lot safer. Alcohol lowers your guard and can lead to taking risks that don't happen when you are alcohol-free.

> *Day 10 for me, double digits and feelin' good. When I started this my partner was pretty unsupportive and against it but today she said, 'Actually, I prefer you not drinking, you're a nicer and better person.' My life is better alcohol-free.*
>
> ***ED***

— You tend to avoid those cringeworthy morning-afters.

— There is a chance to really get to know the person you're out with. From the outset there is no pretence or alcohol-fuelled version of you; it's your authentic self that they're seeing.

— There is something magnetic about being clear-headed when most people around you are looking and sounding worse for wear.

— You win some BIG respect for being on your challenge. It makes you interesting. You will have a story to tell.

— Finally, meeting new people is not all about alcohol and nights out. Being alcohol-free and trying a new activity, such as going to the gym, might lead to a chance meeting.

Or you might get to know someone within a new group you're inspired to join. The options are almost limitless but you can rest assured that feeling and looking great will only lead to more opportunities to meet new and exciting people.

So let's flip the alcohol-single idea on its head. Just imagine how many times a potential soul mate could have crossed your path, yet you missed them in the fog of alcohol. Perhaps that knowing glance or chance conversation was lost to another round. Maybe this alcohol-free adventure will create the spark to make that eye contact, to start the conversation that leads to something special.

ANDY'S STORY

With all the extra time I unearthed, I decided to go back to university part-time. Firstly to finish a degree, then to study for a masters in positive psychology. I also managed to squeeze in the time to qualify as a master practitioner of NLP (Neuro-Linguistic Programming) and become a mindfulness-based awareness coach. On top of all that, I still had time to run a business, enjoy my family, friends and hobbies. What's more, I truly believe that I would have accomplished absolutely none of these achievements if alcohol had still been zapping my time.

GET YOUR TIME BACK

The great philosopher Seneca sums up our relationship with time perfectly when he suggests:

'It is not that we have a short time to live, but that we waste a lot of it.'

Most people would agree that time is our most valuable asset. We only have limited minutes on this planet and the clock is ticking. Once we quit alcohol we realised just how much time it was stealing. The lack of energy, the nights spent chasing drink and the days lost to hangovers meant that there was less and less time for the things – and people – that we loved.

Maybe you're a far more moderate drinker than we used to be, or perhaps you simply don't suffer from hangovers, but we will wager you'll still find a renewed sense of energy once you're alcohol-free, with more time in the day to be productive.

Once alcohol-free we maintained our social bonds yet skipped the silly nights out and hangovers. As our energy came flooding back we started to claw back time. We replaced recovery naps and weekends spent on the couch with early morning bike rides and long-delayed household chores. We were finally able to get out there and live life. By starting our days early, we managed to carve out an extra 2–3 hours a day, which was just the start of our new productivity. This new time was used in various ways – to create OneYearNoBeer, write this book, meditate and exercise, and all before the kids were up. This practice makes a massive difference to our lives today and simply would not exist if hangovers still dominated our mornings.

Since starting my AF journey my weekends are amazing. They start with the local Parkrun on a Saturday morning (including a run there and back) so I have 10,000 steps in the bag before 10am. The rest of the day is then mine to spend time with the hubby, grandkids or my niece. I have so much time and I now spend it really living instead of sleepwalking. Life really is what you make it.

JOANNE

QUALITY TIME

This morning routine was just one aspect of the time advantage. With no hangovers hampering weekends, we started to take up old hobbies and interests as well as create quality family time.

Waking up on a Saturday morning after a great night's sleep, with a clear head, full of vitality and ready for the weekend, is one of life's great joys. This was a major difference from our old alcohol-fuelled life. In theory, a weekend is a weekend, whether you are hungover or not, so we had the same amount of time as before, but being alcohol-free meant we used this time to better effect.

The kicker was that as we reintroduced hobbies and pursued other interests our worlds were no longer just work, stress and staying afloat. Life was getting exciting.

PRODUCTIVITY GOES SKY HIGH

The combination of no hangovers, quality sleep and more time sent our productivity through the roof. We'll say this again and again: one of the greatest achievements in life is performing at your best. As our productivity increased, so did our chances of realising our long-held goals.

In our experience, if you have a desire to get fit, run a marathon, win a promotion, learn a language, take a degree or generally achieve something productive that's been sitting on the back burner for too long, going alcohol-free gives you a massive advantage.

PEAK PERFORMANCE

As we both became more productive at work, we opened the door to a peak performance advantage. We are all in daily competition whether we like it or not. The world moves at such a fast pace that leaders must fend off challengers and challengers must outperform the leaders. At an individual level, there is competition for jobs, followed by competition for pay rises and bonuses. In many ways we are like everyday athletes; we all aim for

After only 70 days, I'm no longer worried about giving in and drinking. I've discovered that I really enjoy AF beer, and it still gives a sense of marking the occasion of finishing a hard day or getting to the end of the week. My husband has joined me on this journey and has only had a few alcoholic drinks while I've remained AF. It's great that we can relax together with our AF beer, talk through our days and make future plans. I suppose in a sense it was never about the alcohol; having a drink was always more about marking an occasion or making time for each other.

LYNETTE

success, facing the best of the best in what we do. We are all professionals in our fields, yet too often we prepare like amateurs.

When we opened our eyes, we began to notice that many of our performance heroes did not drink or drank very little. They had worked it out ahead of the game that in order to perform at their peak, alcohol was not an option.

During an interview on our podcast with the productivity guru Jeff Sanders, we discovered just how powerful a productivity tool being alcohol-free actually is. Jeff has built a career around being productive, yet he still had the odd drink. Like so many of us, this productivity superhero had a blind spot to alcohol. After 30 days alcohol-free his feedback was tremendous:

'I am amazed at the difference being alcohol-free has made. I get another 30 minutes every day that did not exist before, which doesn't sound a lot, but over time this is massive in terms of productivity.'

Wow – one of the world's leading experts on productivity just carved out another 30 minutes every day just from being alcohol-free. Now this is what we're talking about. Forget the wonderful health benefits – if you want to get stuff done, it is clear as day, taking a break from alcohol will help.

RELAX

We both have been guilty of using alcohol as a quick way to de-stress and relax. We won't deny that alcohol can produce those warm fuzzy feelings that help troubles melt away, but the short-term feelings of relaxation are totally undone by the added stress, poor sleep and lethargy that follow the morning after. Short-term gain, long-term pain. That was until our alcohol-free adventures forced us to find other ways to de-stress that actually helped and that did not carry any morning-after consequences.

The simple option was to replace the routine. Swap the beer in the fridge for a really nice alcohol-free alternative. After a long hard day at work, we could still kick back, chill out and crack open a bottle, albeit alcohol-free. This was a great way to relax, yet skip the hangovers and extra morning stress. We also started to experiment with exercise, reading, meditation, cooking, watching TV, writing, listening to music… all of these activities have been proven to reduce stress and help people unwind[3]. The combination of these newfound ways to relax created an upward relaxation spiral. As each day started with less stress and higher energy, we found spare time to attend a yoga class, exercise, meditate and take part in hobbies, which further reduced our stress. Also, as our sleep improved, stress lowered further still. Within a short space of time we created a relaxing existence, all without a drop of alcohol in sight.

There is no one size fits all when it comes to relaxing and de-stressing. The key is to experiment and discover what works for you. Once again, being forced to look for alternatives provided another advantage as

ANDY'S STORY

I am asked on a regular basis to deliver keynotes and people believe that I'm super confident. Just a few months ago my confidence was shot because alcohol had tricked me into believing that without it I had none. Now please don't misunderstand me, I still fear public speaking, but I love the buzz of knowing that I have conquered this particular fear. There is real power in taking on your big confidence challenges with a clear head. This is the stuff that builds a deep confidence.

we discovered many different ways to unwind without alcohol.

We recognise that life is far from perfect and that stress is an inevitable part of our worlds, but by practising these new skills and techniques, we felt better prepared when stressful moments arrived. Those situations that had previously provided an excuse for a skinful were now greeted as a chance to face these obstacles with a clear head. It is amazing the power that comes from dealing with all that life throws at you without the crutch of an alcoholic drink.

I have a new self-confidence where I believe I can do anything I want. An alcohol-free life is full of wonderful and unexpected surprises and increased self-belief, both personally and professionally. I always had grand plans in my head, but that is where they stayed, swamped by a fog that I wasn't worthy or imprisoned by insecurity. This new AF lifestyle has freed me from doubt and I now approach each new day with a newfound energy and zest that means that the future is filled with ambition and I have genuine excitement about what I am capable of…

MARK

Confidence appears in many forms and we were guilty of making the mistake of believing that 'confidence' meant being the centre of attention, being the larger-than-life persona that alcohol created. Whereas in truth, real confidence comes from being your authentic self.

JUST THE RIGHT AMOUNT OF CONFIDENCE

The role alcohol plays in our lives is summed up nicely by the wedding speech scenario. Very often this is a moment many of us dread. A survey found that public speaking is our second biggest fear[4] (death is number one). The wedding speech is a great moment in one's life, but it can also present a massive confidence challenge. At weddings all over the land someone is playing the alcohol = confidence game. The rules are simple: you try to drink the perfect amount to feel some fake confidence, but not so much that you end up slurring your words. Or, worst of all, you don't drink enough and you have to make the speech SOBER.

GET YOUR REAL CONFIDENCE BACK

We both worried what would happen to our confidence without Dutch courage. The quick answer? It came flooding back. This classic alcohol trick was so evident it was almost palpable. What it pretended to offer with one hand it was taking away with the other. Admittedly, it was hard at first to mingle socially without the crutch of alcohol, but over time we could feel a different confidence rising.

The confidence that comes from going alcohol-free is deep and long lasting.

Taking on confidence challenges with a clear head provides a massive life advantage. Just imagine having the deep confidence to take on a big moment like this with ease.

WHAT YOU DO MATTERS

One of the most powerful indicators of well-being is believing that what you do matters. As our alcohol-free adventure progressed we found a powerful confidence building and could see that our actions made a difference. We realised that through our own efforts we could go against the grain to create the lives we wanted. This snowballed into a proactive confidence that propelled us to take on more and more well-being and life challenges. For example, our diets started to evolve because we knew deep down that we could change our habits and our worlds.

As our confidence came flooding back we discovered a deep belief in ourselves that Dutch courage couldn't touch.

THE WARM-UP

We totally appreciate that, for some, taking a break from alcohol appears pretty simple, while for others, like us, it was a major undertaking. It felt so big at times that the enormity of the task ahead almost prevented us from starting.

For those who don't suffer the dreaded hangover, or just have them from time to time, this challenge will motivate you to unlock the ultimate healthy lifestyle. Even the smallest gains – from improved sleep to extra productivity – will make a massive difference to your world. Through our successes and failures we stumbled upon wisdom that improved our outlook far beyond simply quitting alcohol.

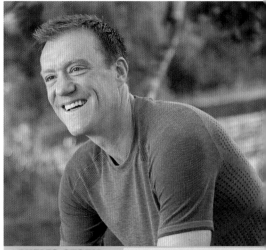

ANDY'S STORY

I can't tell you how many times I slipped up having made a rational decision to stop drinking.

I would find myself in a social situation full of good intentions not to drink. Then as I approached the bar with my healthy option at the forefront of my mind, I would suddenly smell the lager, hear the clatter of glasses and sense the heady ambiance. A question would cut through the beer-soaked air. A question that I had been asked a thousand times before:

What do you want to drink, sir? Erm... Pint of lager, please!

WHAT? How did that happen? Where did my rational choice go?

When a slip-up such as this occurs, we often feel embarrassed and berate ourselves: 'I obviously don't have any willpower,' 'I can't do this,' 'I am not like those other willpower heroes,' 'I'm a failure,' 'My genes are faulty.' Worse still, a belief grows that you might have that disease they talk about. OMG, am I addicted to alcohol?

Unfortunately, the easiest way to cover up this self-proclaimed lack of follow-through is to not follow through, and to give up by sweeping the perceived lack of willpower under the carpet. We tell ourselves, 'I will just keep drinking like everyone else because the safest place to hide is in the crowd.' The result of this mindset is that an opportunity for positive change is lost because of a misunderstanding of how the brain really works.

The next problem with an unaddressed slip-up is that it can trigger the 'What the hell' effect. This cognitive licence leads to mass overindulgence and was first discovered by Janet Polivy, of the dieting world, when she noticed that many of her clients were falling off the wagon in style every time they slipped up[5]. Once they felt that the diet was blown, the clients triggered the 'What the hell' effect, telling themselves, 'I may as well eat 10 cakes now that I have eaten the one.' Rather than one slip-up being treated as exactly that, it seemed to open the floodgates to days of overindulgence.

It's exactly the same with alcohol. We tell ourselves, 'I slipped up and had a glass of wine. Oh well, I may as well finish the bottle.'

So what's happening here with all these slip-ups?

Professor Steve Peters, the legendary psychologist behind the Team Sky and Great Britain Olympic cycling successes, describes our brains using a human versus chimp analogy. Peters suggests the limbic part of our brain, which stores our habits and routines, is like our inner chimp. Just like a real-world chimp, it is much stronger than the 'human' rational part of our brain and in a straight fight will always win[6].

The trick is to use your rational brain to train this inner chimp to want the right things. Once trained, you will have a powerful ally and your chances of creating positive change will be greatly enhanced. The aim behind the OYNB habit-change system is to train your inner chimp and to reprogramme the limbic part of your brain to support the healthy habit of taking a break from alcohol.

It's these subtle mindset shifts that will make all the difference to your challenge. By simply learning about how our brains work when it comes to habits, we can take all the power out of these situations and stay on track to creating lasting habit-change.

Understanding why slip-ups happen can help us avoid the 'What the hell' effect. You need a system to take a break from booze, because without help you might miss out on the chance to create the life you always wanted.

> *‚WITHOUT HELP YOU MIGHT MISS OUT ON THE CHANCE TO CREATE THE LIFE YOU ALWAYS WANTED.‚*

During our lives we are faced with many trials, stressors, dilemmas and obstacles, yet our brains and bodies want the easy route. We don't like trouble or breaks from the norm. Our instincts want to proliferate our genes into the next generation then check out – job done. The path of least resistance is an attractive option, but the problem with this path is that it's a terrible teacher. When we turn away from difficult situations we miss the chance to learn.

BEHIND THE MOUNTAINS ARE MORE MOUNTAINS

Let's not kid ourselves that overcoming our biggest obstacles will make the rest vanish. As you break through your barriers, more appear, but each one you conquer equips you to face the next trial with even more strength. Every time you'll learn something new about yourself. Every time you'll develop strength, wisdom and perspective, until all that's left is the best version of you.

So if you are ready to take on the challenge, remember the maxim 'the obstacle is the way.' These five little words have had a massive impact on our lives and we hope they help you, too.

At this point there is not much to do apart from get started, because the magic is in the doing when it comes to this challenge.

Before we kick things off, let's get warmed up for the exciting adventure ahead by answering a few of the questions and concerns that you might have.

I would love to start, but I have a birthday, wedding, stag do, office party, [fill in blank] coming up …
When people consider a challenge like this the first thing they do is look at their diary and proclaim, 'Oh, I can't start now because of the wedding, hen, birthday, office party…' The thing is, there will always be some major event on the horizon. Our lives are so busy that a clear path rarely exists. The key point here is that these events provide some of best alcohol-free moments. Rather than being a reason to put off starting the challenge, these social occasions are the best reason to start.

There is something powerful about enjoying the office party alcohol-free or dancing sober at a wedding. When you tackle these events with a clear head and enjoy them, you start to smash many of your limiting beliefs around alcohol. There is a real sense that you can still have a great social life and skip the debilitating hangovers. Once you take on a big occasion, the little ones are a walk in the park. It might seem hard to fathom right now, but trust us, it's true, and the best part is when you wake up the next day full of beans while your friends are suffering with hangovers.

I will start tomorrow
You may have heard the story about the guy who is 100 per cent determined to quit alcohol. He decides there and then that tomorrow is the day that he will definitely stop drinking for good. So he finds a piece

of paper and writes in large bold letters: 'Tomorrow I will stop drinking alcohol – forever.'

Before he goes to bed he pins the message on his bedside wall, so that on waking he will be instantly reminded of the promise he made. That night he sleeps like a baby. On waking the first thing he sees is the sign and reads the message aloud. 'Tomorrow I will stop drinking alcohol – forever.'

Don't wait for a tomorrow that never comes, put an X on today and make this Day 1 of your alcohol-free adventure.

The final question – why do I need help to give up alcohol in the first place?

Surely all of us could, if we wanted to, just make a rational decision to stop drinking and that's it, job done. The beer can't jump out of the glass into our mouths – or can it?

Wouldn't it be great if life was really like this? If it were, there would be no need for New Year's resolutions that we break five minutes after midnight. How boring would life be if we made our lists and stuck to them! Part of the excitement and challenge of living is overcoming desires, fears and failures in order to build a world that thrives.

So before we talk habit change systems and how we will help you take a break from alcohol, let's answer the question above by answering another burning question.

What happens if I slip up?

A major lesson we discovered on a personal level and when helping thousands of others change their habits is that slip-ups are ok.

We need to be very clear about this: we do not encourage slip-ups or offer tactical breaks. The reality is that we often slip up, but not for the reason most of us believe. The science suggests our digressions have less to do with willpower, as we commonly think, and more to do with psychological and social conditioning. In short, we are what our habits dictate.

Let us explain: we all slip up from time to time and this is perfectly normal. Unfortunately, there is a tendency to fall into the trap of believing we are perfectly rational human beings – when we're not. The majority of us believe that we simply make a rational decision and that's all there is to it. If we fail to act on this rational choice, then we obviously lack the willpower required.

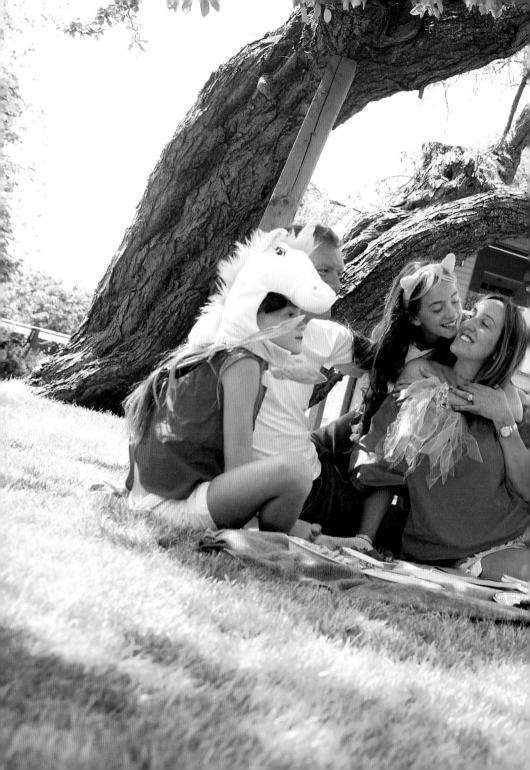

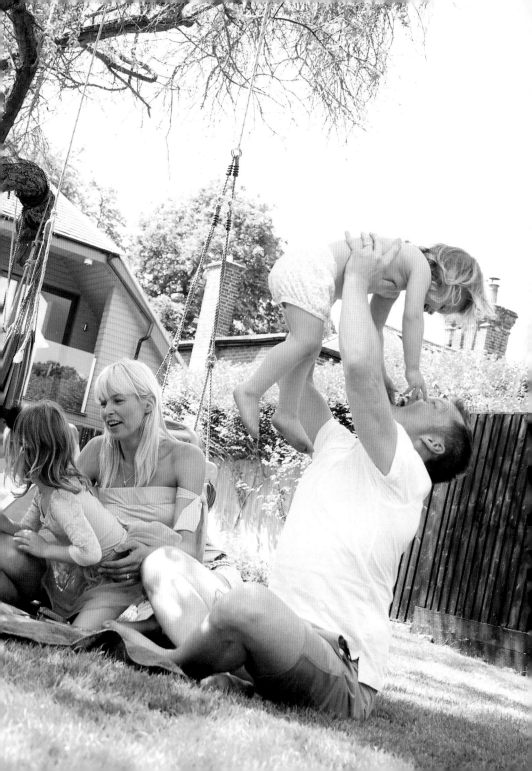

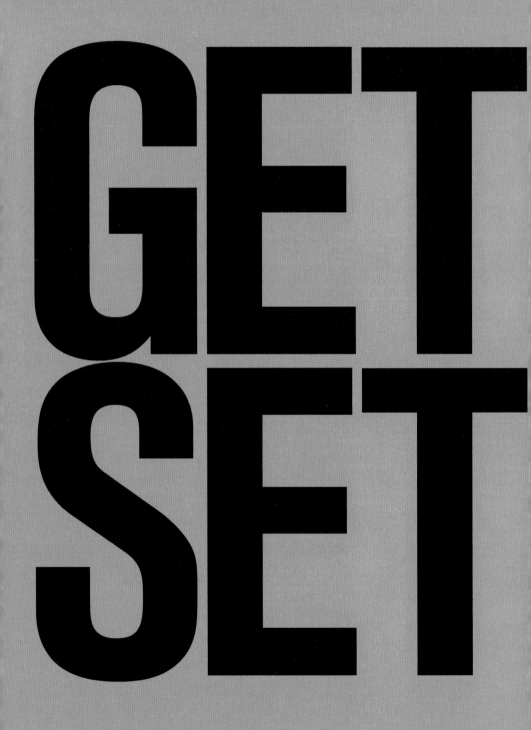

THE MEND HABIT-CHANGE SYSTEM

We have broken up this challenge into 28 days of daily support, tips, tricks, hacks and techniques to make your challenge as enjoyable as possible. Each day's learning sits neatly within our unique habit-change system that we call MEND.

The power of the MEND system is in the doing, so let's start with a brief overview. MEND stands for the four elements that make up our powerful habit-change system:

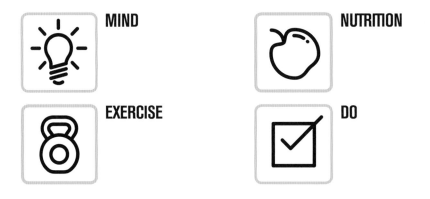

MIND

NUTRITION

EXERCISE

DO

The MEND system is designed to work at the root of our psychological and social conditioning. The ultimate aim of this system is to help people build such a vibrant alcohol-free life that the thought of going back to hangovers, lethargy and regret is simply not an option. In doing so, we rewire our brains to support these new and empowering healthy habits.

At this point a total mindset shift takes place and the battle is won. You no longer want to drink alcohol because it's not part of the amazing, healthy, vibrant lifestyle you've created. Alcohol is no longer something you're giving up, but a threat to your dreams and goals. At this point, you will no longer see yourself as a drinker, but someone who is loving life alcohol-free.

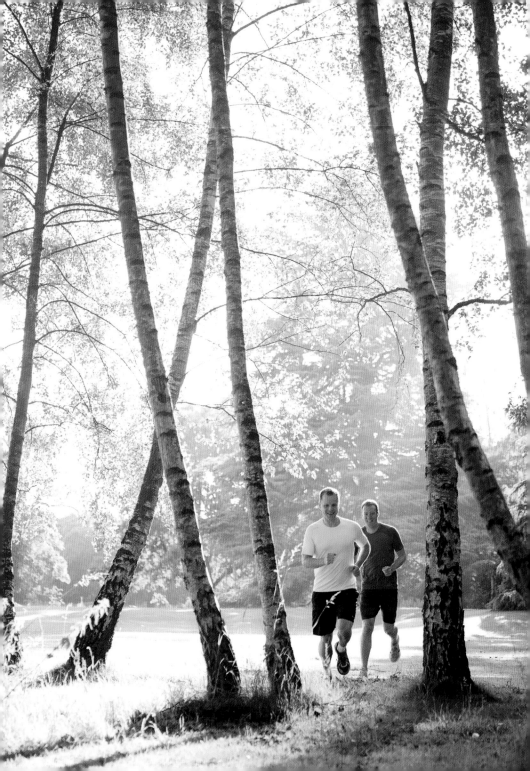

HOW THE MEND SYSTEM WORKS

 MIND
To effect lasting habit-change we need to reprogramme our minds to support these new empowering habits. At OYNB our mission is to search for the best ways to make this happen. The techniques and skills we introduce come from the fields of positive psychology, sports psychology, Neuro-Linguistic Programming (NLP), mindfulness, behavioural science, the science of habit-change and, finally, a large dollop of our own experience. The aim of the game is to unlock our minds and replace unhelpful habits such as drinking alcohol with healthy, empowering alternative habits.

Throughout the book you will find techniques and skills that are designed to retrain your brain and to support you on this challenge. Positive psychology, the science behind well-being, will improve your overall mental well-being, which builds the foundations of habit-change. Mindfulness is used to shine a spotlight on your subconscious routines, from where you can make a conscious choice about which routines you want to change. The science of habit-change is then used to help break the bad ones and promote the good. NLP provides many wonderful examples of visualisation techniques to help you mentally rehearse these new habits. All of these MIND skills will help you smash this challenge and change your habits around alcohol for good.

 EXERCISE
Exercise is a wonderful conduit to habit-change. Firstly, exercise is still one of the best physical and mental health interventions on the planet[7]. Any move to enhance well-being is welcomed, so exercise is a great place to start. From Day 1 we will encourage you to book yourself into a physical challenge that is just beyond your current capabilities. Also, when exercise is combined with the loss of alcoholic calories and better nutrition, people's bodies start to change, which is a wonderful motivator.

To be clear, this is not all about running marathons or HIIT (high intensity interval training) sessions. Gentle exercise such as walking and Tai Chi are also excellent conduits to habit-change.

The major reason why exercise is such a brilliant habit-change tool is that it helps build self-confidence so that you feel you can make a positive difference in your life. It is this mindset of belief that will help power you to lasting positive change.

NUTRITION

The ultimate healthy lifestyle combines the trilogy of mind, exercise and diet. We are what we eat. When most people think about quitting alcohol the last thing they consider is changing their diet to help. This is where we think differently. We treat habit-change as an athlete would treat a race. The difference between success and failure is so small that we want to establish every marginal gain we can to add up to major, lasting and positive habit-change. What we eat helps drive the mind, provides the energy to exercise and keeps our willpower reserves high. For this reason, quality nutrition is key to habit-change.

During Day 9 we dive deep into more specific nutritional information. We have layered various nutritional tips and facts throughout the book, from supplement advice to tasty alcohol-free drinks to wow your party guests.

DO

We can all talk a good game but until we act on these ideas, they are just that – ideas. Our aim is to get people out of their habitual comfort zones to DO stuff – take on physical challenges, learn new skills and socialise without alcohol, and DO all those things that an alcohol-free lifestyle promotes. It is 'action' that brings this challenge to life.

The combination of learning new habit-change techniques and making a first-hand experience of life alcohol-free helps solidify new and healthy habits. For example, when you do stuff and take on social events alcohol-free you start to bust those long-held myths. The specific habit-change techniques and skills that you will do also help create new healthy habits.

There is a great saying: 'neurons that fire together wire together', and by creating new experiences and trying new skills you will build habitual pathways that will lead to lasting positive habit-change.

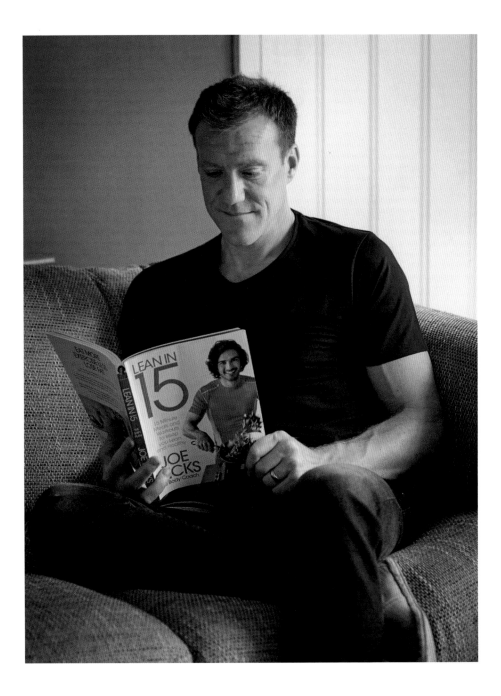

PUTTING IT ALL TOGETHER

All the MEND elements are designed specifically to break unwanted habits while promoting preferred ones. Hopefully you have noticed a running theme here: in order to crack the alcohol habit we will subtly build new healthy, empowering ones. This creates a win–win scenario where not only do you give yourself the best chance at lasting change, but you also unlock a vibrant, healthy lifestyle!

To be clear, we know we don't have all the answers. We are learning every day from our members which techniques work and which ones are less effective. There is a constant and neverending quest for improvement, which is a challenge we both relish.

Hopefully by now you are full of excitement, pumped and ready to kick-start this life-enhancing challenge. So let's get practical. The time for talk is over – you are warmed up and ready to go. Let your 28-day alcohol-free challenge begin!

YOUR TOOLBOX

'Fail to prepare, prepare to fail.'
SAS mantra

Our mission is to help you prepare, prepare and then prepare some more. You are now an alcohol-free athlete getting ready for the race of a lifetime.

Like most things in life, the more effort you put in, the more you will get out. Throw yourself into the exercises, try out the tips and push yourself to experience the different techniques. View this challenge like any other – from a triathlon to a mud race. The ideas that follow are your very own alcohol-free toolbox. You can constantly refer to these discoveries for extra motivation, inspiration and tools to make this challenge a fantastic experience.

At the end of your challenge you will be able to look yourself in the mirror knowing that you have experienced life without alcohol. It is at this point that you can decide whether you want to continue with the challenge, drink occasionally in full control or never drink again. The choice, as always, will be yours.

Good luck! We will be with you every step of the way.

Andy and Ruari

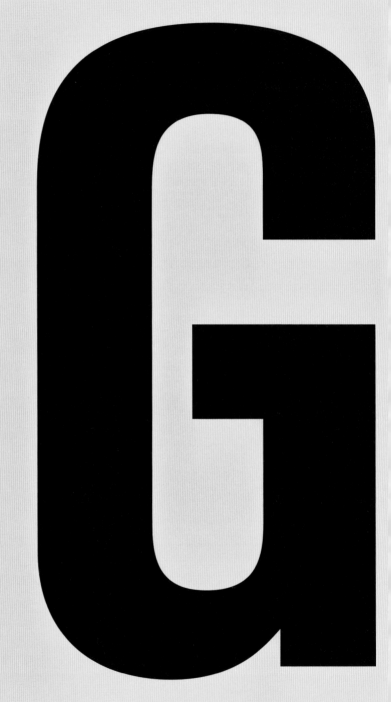

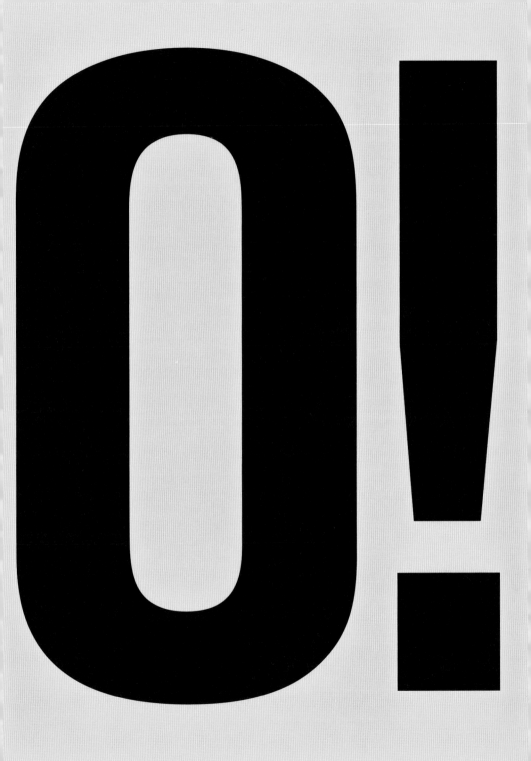

THE 28-DAY CHAMPION CHALLENGE

For every day of the challenge you'll have a mix of different things to think about or put into action, tying in to the MEND system. Each new day builds on the preceding ones, so by the end of the challenge you'll have a whole arsenal of different strategies for putting alcohol in its place.

Before you start we would like you to do two things:

1. Take a photo or photos of what you look like today. Keep these snaps where you can refer back to them in a few weeks to see the difference in your eyes, face and body.

2. Fill out our quick progress tracker below. Give yourself a rating out of 10 for each of the categories, with 1 being a poor rating and 10 being amazing.

Better yet, record your responses so you can track your changes over time at **members.oneyearnobeer.com/Test/Week1**

QUICK PROGRESS TRACKER	
HAPPINESS	/10
MOTIVATION	/10
PRODUCTIVITY	/10
SLEEP	/10
ENERGY	/10
TIME	/10
EXERCISE	/10
OVERALL SCORE	**/70**

Note: we will ask you to fill out this tracker once a week until the end of your challenge so you can easily see how far you have come in such a short space of time.

Remember, you don't have to do this alone. Sign up to www.oneyearnobeer.com and join a vibrant community of people just like you. This group is being talked about as one of the best on the net and they will support you and inspire you to challenge glory. You will also receive daily emails with everything you need to know.

3. Track your progress online and take the quick online well-being survey: oneyearnobeer.com/start-survey

Ok, it's game on. Let's do this!

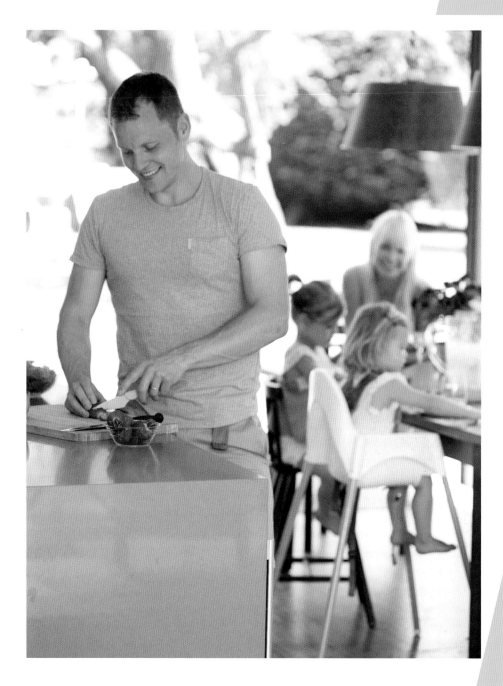

WEEK 1 HABITS

Your first week is so important, and the effort you put in now will set you up for the rest of this challenge. As the alcohol leaves your system, your motivation and productivity will come rushing back. By the end of this first week you will start to feel many of the advantages of being alcohol-free, such as more time, energy and emotional fitness, which will propel you into 'willpower' Week 2.

In these early days you might also notice the benefits of a deep restorative night's sleep, although for some, as the alcohol departs your system, you might feel a little restless at night. We will share with you the best way to get off to sleep without a drop of alcohol. You will also learn from the masters how to improve the quality of your sleep.

During the course of this week you will discover more about the science of habits, and we will show you how to break your bad ones and enhance the good. You will also need to book a physical challenge, and we'll teach you how to deal with those people who just don't understand why you're on this alcohol-free adventure.

Finally, during this first week we will show you what you need to know, when you need to know it.

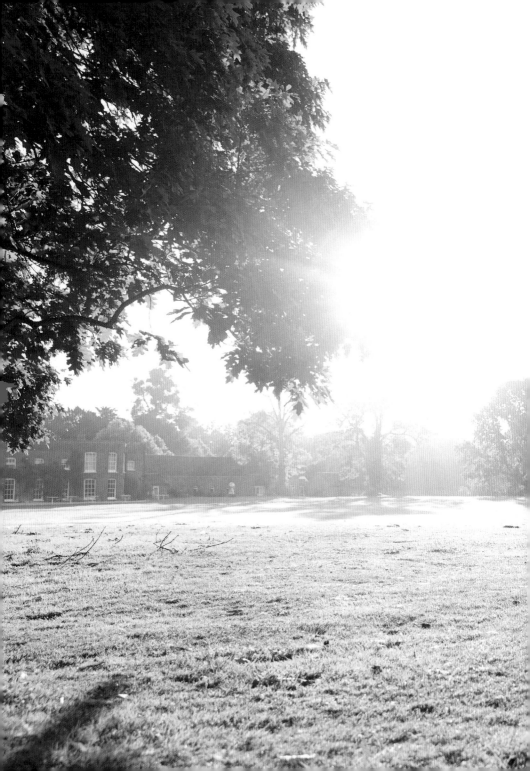

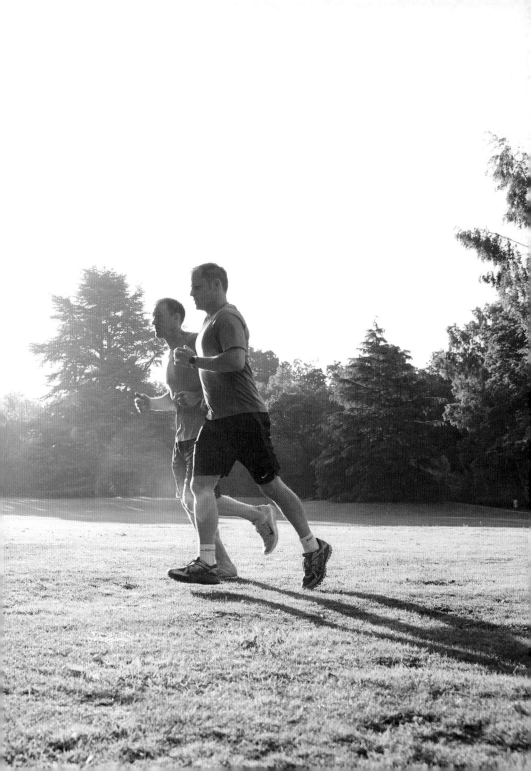

DAY 1

‘*WHEN YOU FIND YOURSELF ON THE SIDE OF THE MAJORITY, IT IS TIME TO PAUSE AND REFLECT*’
MARK TWAIN [8]

WHY ARE YOU HERE?

Let's kick off this challenge by writing down all the reasons why you are here. Ask yourself, why have you decided to take this challenge? What will it offer you? What will you gain by completing 28 days alcohol-free?

We want you to dig deep and make this a visceral experience. Really try to get to the bottom of why, exactly, you are here. A great tool to help you to go deeper is to ask yourself each time you think you are finished, 'and what else?' Think of as many reasons as you can and let your mind run free. There are no wrong or right answers! You might notice that many habit-change techniques in this book seem simple, such as the idea of making notes. But don't be fooled, these approaches pack a powerful punch. There is much research to suggest that the simple act of writing down your thoughts and emotions is good for you[9]. The cathartic act of releasing your inner ideas is often enough to trigger many well-being benefits.

The reason we ask you to note down these thoughts is to provide a constant reminder of why you're here, both during the good times and the tough times.

It appears we have short memories when it comes to going alcohol-free, and we have noticed people tend to trip up when they begin to drop their guard, often around Week 2. In many cases, this happens as their energy comes flooding back and they feel so good that they forget all the reasons why they started this challenge in the first place.

WHY ARE YOU HERE?
Right now, in this moment, while the memories are fresh, perform this exercise. Ideally, go old school and use pen and paper, but an iPad, laptop or whatever suits you will work, too.

Take five minutes to list all the reasons why you decided to take this challenge. Make sure that your reasons are kept somewhere handy so you can refer to them as much as possible during your challenge. This list will keep you motivated and will also remind you why you are here when you need that nudge.

Some members stick their reasons onto the bathroom mirror or put motivational Post-it notes on their computer screens. Get creative! This is your world, do whatever works for you.

If you need help, here is some inspiration from your fellow alcohol-free challenge participants as to why they are here:

'To be able to go out and then remember the conversation the next day.' **Karen**

'To be more patient.' **Emma**

'I want to be a better dad.' **Mark**

'My mission is to run a marathon and I know this challenge will help me achieve that.' **David**

'To realize new ambitions, such as being a published writer.' **Liz**

RESTOCK THE FRIDGE

For those who like to drink predominantly at home, social pressure is less of a factor, which is great, but this can mean more pitfalls.

Firstly, the home bar never shuts and it serves generous measures. Also, there is no wait for the first social occasion to test your alcohol-free skills; it's game on from the second you start this challenge. So let's prepare you for this hurdle from the off.

Research has shown that when faced with our desires we find it much harder to make the best choices. For example, office workers ate over four times more sweets when they were moved from opaque containers placed 2m away to see-through containers put right on their desks[10], while children living in areas surrounded by fast-food outlets are more likely to be overweight[11].

In these early days, don't feel that you have to be a willpower super hero. If most of your drinking is done at home, try to remove temptation. This might sound over the top, but let's not forget you have been psychologically programmed for a long time to behave in a certain way. It will take time to overwrite these old habits with new healthier ones. We have all been there; the

wine monster makes a sudden appearance and we go looking for a drink. When there is no ready supply available, the craving subsides – panic over, slip-up avoided.

 REMOVE AND RESTOCK
So today, where possible, remove temptation. We understand you might be throwing money down the drain, but by not buying alcohol regularly, as you did before, you will save much more than you throw away.

Next, restock the fridge with some nice alcohol-free alternatives for when the booze monster strikes. If you want to replace like for like, buy a selection of alcohol-free beers or wine – they are improving all the time and taste pretty good. Also, alcohol-free spirits such as Seedlip are injecting new life into mocktails, making tasty lookalikes even easier to make.

'I cleared out the fridge and put in a mixture of alcohol-free beers. I was amazed at the selection and I am going to try one per night during this first week.' **Lenny**

Putting these small measures in place at the start of your challenge will make a massive difference over the next three weeks.

BUY YOURSELF SOME TIME

If you open the fridge and are faced with a cold beer, wait five minutes to try to avoid temptation. Tell yourself that you can have it, if you really want it, in five minutes. We know this is easier said than done, for all the reasons already mentioned, but this little break will make a big difference. The extra time slows the dopamine rush (your craving chemicals), giving you the space to make a choice that fits your goals.

IS IT OK TO DRINK ALCOHOL-FREE ALTERNATIVES THAT CONTAIN A SMALL AMOUNT OF ALCOHOL?

This is a question we are asked all the time and the answer is a big yes. The whole aim of this challenge is to change your relationship with alcohol, and alcohol-free alternatives are a great way to help this process. Some will contain minimal amounts of alcohol, such as 0.5 per cent, but in reality this volume of alcohol is so small it will not hinder the process of change, and that's all that matters.

USE THE EXCUSE

At this early stage you are still programmed with the alcohol habit. Over the next weeks we will replace this habit with healthy empowering ones.

Let's face it, alcohol is the only drug in the world that when you give it up, people berate you. It's sad but true, so unless you have a decent excuse for not drinking, your rubber arm will be twisted. We created this challenge to provide the excuse you need to get out of the alcohol-free starter's blocks in full view of family, friends and colleagues. Many people love a challenge. It seems

everyone is taking part in a mud race or running a marathon these days. Going alcohol-free is a massive challenge for most – and one that deserves respect. So we thought we'd add 'not drinking' to the list of these favourite challenges.

'Do you want a drink?'
'No, I'm on a 28-day alcohol-free challenge. I thought it would be a real test and I have to say I am enjoying it.'
'OK, fair enough.'

As this movement grows, more people will hear about this challenge, which will make it easier for those taking part. Our dream is that one day this 28-day adventure will be a totally normal reason to take a break.

SUPPLEMENT HELP?

More evidence is needed, but if you're struggling with alcohol cravings, a supplement of glutamine (stocked by most health foods stores and also available online) could be worth a try. In a study back in the 1950s, a gram of glutamine per day given in divided portions with meals decreased both the desire to drink and anxiety levels. In a later study a combination supplement including glutamine and a multivitamin also reduced withdrawal symptoms and decreased stress. Always check with your doctor before taking supplements if you're on other medications or have a medical condition.

DAY 2

'THE GOLDEN RULE OF HABIT-CHANGE: YOU CAN'T EXTINGUISH A BAD HABIT, YOU CAN ONLY CHANGE IT'

CHARLES DUHIGG [12]

THE HABIT LOOP

First and foremost, the aim of this challenge is to break a small, tiny, minuscule habit: drinking alcohol. For the vast majority that's all it is – a habit – and habits can be broken.

Our dream is to not only break the habits that are holding you back, but to also promote and create healthy new ones. But for now, let's focus on the number one bad habit: booze.

THE HABIT LOOP

Our brains love habits because they save precious energy. For this reason, wherever possible, our grey matter will look to create routines so it does not have to waste energy thinking about these actions. These habits, from brushing your teeth to riding a bike, can then run on autopilot.

This is great for healthy habits, but it's a problem for the bad ones. This is why awareness is so important for habit-change, because it brings our subconscious routines into the light of consciousness. Once we are aware of our habits – good and bad – we can start to promote the good and break the bad.

Science tells us that a habit is formed when four elements come together:

Cue

There is a trigger or cue that starts the habit process.

Routine

This is the action that is played out.

Reward

At the end of the routine is the reward.

Craving

The reward drives the whole loop as you crave its pleasures.

As long as there is a reward at the end of the loop that your brain likes, it does not question the routine, it just gets on with it. This is how problems start. For example, once a bad habit is formed, the brain happily stops thinking about it, leaving us with routines that are performed on autopilot below our conscious radar, which, if left unchecked, can do serious damage without us realising.

Imagine your brain as an old vinyl record. Each time you repeat a process, the record groove gets slightly deeper, making it even easier for the needle to find its way back to that part of the song. Over time these grooves become so deep that trying to move the needle is tricky.

We will cover each section of the habit loop in more detail as you progress through the challenge, but for now let's take a quick peek at the process as a whole.

STEP ONE:
WHAT'S YOUR TRIGGER?

Our lives are so busy that trying to find a trigger amongst the noise of our day is extremely difficult. Once again, science is here to help – almost all triggers are created within the following five categories[13]:

— **Location**
— **Time**
— **Emotional state**
— **Other people**
— **Preceding action – this could include activities such as lighting a cigarette.**

QUICK TRIGGER FINDER

The next time you experience a craving, use the five categories above as a guide to help uncover your trigger. It could be any one of the five or a combination of a few. The key is to uncover as many of these triggers as possible. Note them down and analyse the findings until you fully understand what's promoting these feelings.

Examples from OYNB members:

Darren

Location: Sitting at the desk
Time: 1 p.m.
Emotional state: Bored
Other people: Colleagues – also bored
Preceding action: WhatsApp from colleague – he is going for a quick one

Clare

Location: Home
Time: 7 p.m.
Emotional state: Stressed
Other people: Partner
Preceding action: He calls wine o'clock

Once you know your triggers it's time to discover the reward you crave.

STEP TWO:
WHAT REWARD IS DRIVING THE HABIT?

Now let's take some time to consider what's driving the habit loop. Is it the social interaction with your colleagues that you crave? Or could it be a misguided attempt at stress relief?

Often the reward driving a habit loop is totally unrelated to the habit itself. For example, having beers after work might be an attempt to relieve boredom or to be seen as part of the 'gang' rather than a craving for the alcohol itself.

This is a key concept to grasp because if you can identify the reward that's driving the habit, you can then create various options to achieve this reward without alcohol.

REWARD FINDER

Jot down all the potential rewards that might be driving your drinking habit. Try to uncover if the reward you seek is something other than the alcohol itself.

STEP THREE:
CHANGE YOUR ROUTINE AND
BREAK BAD HABITS

The best way to break bad habits is to dress them up as new ones. This is the genius of habit-change: once you understand your trigger and reward, all you have to do is change the routine. The loop remains but you trick your brain into substituting a new empowering habit for one that's holding you back. The grooves of the record are the same but the song is different. Beautiful.

EXAMPLES
Routine
Swap the alcoholic beer for an alcohol-free alternative.

Routine
Instead of pouring a glass of wine, de-stress with a run or a five-minute meditation.

You get the idea – keep experimenting with your world until you create routines that support your goals.

CELEBRATE HABIT-HACK SUCCESS
Finally, each time you hack a habit, reward your efforts. The heightened awareness that you're bringing into your life gives you back control and this is worth celebrating. Why not treat yourself with some of the extra cash that you're saving? The choice, as always, is yours, but do make sure you congratulate yourself and acknowledge your achievement.

HABIT HACK
For the rest of the day, be on the lookout for your habits, good and bad. Make a note of them and see if you can figure out the trigger, routine and reward. This exercise is not exclusive to alcohol; aim to notice any habits – from eating cake to biting your nails. The key is to gain experience using the habit loop.

So every time you're tempted by the cake, drink, cigarette or any other type of habit, take 30 seconds and walk through these steps:

— **What's the trigger?**
— **What reward am I seeking?**
— **What routine can I put in its place?**
— **How can I celebrate hacking this habit?**

The more you perform this groundwork the easier your challenge will be. It's really that simple.

THREE SIMPLE WAYS TO RESIST
AN ALCOHOL URGE

1. Eat regularly and don't skip meals. Now is not the time to try a fasting or low-carb diet (see Healthy Carbs on page 100).

2. Stay hydrated – feeling thirsty on a hot day can amplify the craving for a beer.

3. Have a 'go-to' beverage that you can enjoy when those around you are having an alcoholic drink – but watch how many calories and how much sugar it contains.

WINE O'CLOCK

We talk a lot about the social pressure that surrounds alcohol, but we do fully appreciate that there are those who prefer to drink at home rather than out in a group. While this negates some of the social pressure, it does mean that you will have to quickly replace your routines with other non-alcohol-based ones to resist succumbing to temptation.

Perhaps you could consider keeping busy during these early days and spending less time at home? For example, take an exercise class after work or go to the cinema. If this is not possible, make extra time to work through the habit loop to ensure you have identified all your triggers and have a selection of healthy routines ready to replace your old drinking routines. Finally, make sure the fridge is restocked (see page 54) and that you have alternatives ready in case the wine monster rears its head.

MYTH BUSTER –
WILL I BE BORING?

Being labelled as boring was one of our biggest alcohol-free fears. What would happen to fun-time Andy and Ruari? Would we be replaced by total bore-offs? It seems silly, but this fear is often what prevents people from taking a break from drinking.

Like most drinkers, we had our repertoire of drunken stories that we carried around like old war medals. We have to admit that some of them are pretty funny on the surface, but underneath they reveal a worrying truth: alcohol alters body and mind, and usually not for the better.

We both knew that if we kept up the alcohol-fuelled revelry, our loved ones, bodies and jobs would all eventually suffer. Yet the thought of going alcohol-free still had us worried.

We were fooled into believing that alcohol alone was bringing enjoyment to our lives, when this was totally untrue. The years of psychological conditioning had wrongly associated alcohol with having a good time, being funny, giving us courage and helping us relax. We had built a belief system that said, 'Life without alcohol would be boring', when this was totally false.

We decided to make a list of what boring meant to us, so that we could discover why on earth alcohol seemed to be the litmus test for fun.

BORING =

— Wasting a whole day on a hangover

— Having no energy to enjoy life

— Feeling unhappy with last night's drinking

— Repeating oneself over and over

— Not listening to a word anyone says during a conversation

— Getting all emotional over nothing

— Eating terrible food

— Not exercising.

FUN =

— Having the energy to get outside and maximise life

— Feeling refreshed the day after the night before

— Having the extra time to pursue hobbies and interests that we love

— Really listening to friends and enjoying deep conversation

— Creating a vibrant social life that is not fixated on alcohol

— Exercising on a daily basis

— Feeling the mental clarity to perform at our best in the office and at home.

When we looked at our boring list, almost all the items were related to or caused by alcohol. So it's time to bust the boring myth, because taking a break from alcohol is anything but boring.

Perhaps make your own list of all the things that you consider boring and all those things you believe are fun. See where alcohol fits in, and bust the boring myth.

DAY 3

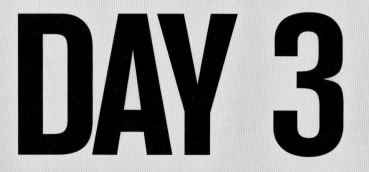

"IF YOU MOVE ENOUGH, YOUR MUSCLES CHANGE AND GROW. SO DOES YOUR MIND. THE BRAIN INITIATES MOVEMENT.

BUT IT IS, IN ITS TURN, REMADE BY MOVEMENT. NEW CELLS ARE BORN; NEW VESSELS SPROUT.

THE SAME PROCESS OPERATES BODY-WIDE. NO CELL IN YOUR BODY IS UNAFFECTED BY MOTION. YOUR VERY DNA IS CHANGED"

GRETCHEN REYNOLDS [14]

LET'S GET PHYSICAL

BOOK A PHYSICAL CHALLENGE

Ok, we know you have just started a challenge and here we are, asking you to book another one. But this is what being alcohol-free is all about – getting out there and doing stuff. We have discovered that exercise is a key part of creating lasting habit-change. Why is that, you might ask?

Firstly, exercise is still the number one well-being pill, and research suggests that exercise builds confidence while enhancing both physical and mental health[15]. Our view of habit-change is simple: if you can build a healthy, vibrant, thriving lifestyle on the back of this alcohol-free challenge, thoughts of throwing this away on hangovers will not be an option. Our aim, therefore, is to not only help you to stop drinking alcohol, but for you to build a healthy lifestyle while also helping you towards the goals you always dreamed of.

Another bonus of creating an exercise challenge is that it provides focus and something to aim for. Once you stop drinking you will be flooded with extra time and energy. Very often there is a need to channel this into something positive. Furthermore, the combination of fewer alcohol calories and exercise can help your body to change shape and look fitter. This often leads to compliments on your healthy appearance, which increases your motivation to stay on your chosen path. Finally, taking on a physical challenge provides a deep confidence that what you do makes a difference. This is such a powerful mental shift and can lead to a whole

host of other well-being benefits. Once you discover that you can change almost anything in your life, you will reach your goals, improve your diet and achieve your dreams.

So this next bit is pretty straightforward. Book a physical challenge of your choice with a start date set towards the end or after your challenge period. This challenge could be a half-hour walk, 5k Parkrun, mud race, bike ride or even a marathon. The choice is yours. To be clear, the type of physical challenge or distance you choose to do irrelevant, because everyone is so different.

There is only one thing you should remember, though: the challenge should be something that pushes you beyond what you are capable of right now.

Note: If you work in a very physical job, as some of our members do, swap this physical challenge with a mental one. Perhaps challenge yourself to learn a language or take an exam. The idea is the same; you need to push yourself beyond your current capabilities.

You will be amazed at what you can achieve with your new body, mind and confidence, so pick something demanding. Do this today.

There are no limits, but please do something that means you push yourself.
Challenge ideas from our members:

- **5k run**
- **Swimathon**
- **Long-distance bike ride**
- **Run a marathon**
- **Hiking and climbing**
- **Tough Mudder and various other obstacle races**
- **Charity night walk.**

GROUP CHALLENGES

Why not join the OYNB team on one of our group challenges? All of these particular challenges have been selected specifically because they can be completed by people with all levels of basic fitness. No one comes last and no one gets a shiny medal for winning; we stay with the group and we help those who need it. This is a team challenge and we love them! The best part of it is – we get to meet you. Check out our website www.oneyearnobeer.com for the latest group challenge.

 COMING OUT OF THE ALCOHOL CLOSET
When you first come out of the booze closet not everyone is going to jump for joy at the new you. It's a shame, but it's true. It could be your best friend, partner or boss, but there will always be someone who simply doesn't get it.

Experiences with alcohol can be highly subjective. For example, when you tell someone who drinks in moderation about your challenge, they might not understand your perspective. They might offer pearls of wisdom such as, 'Why don't you just drink less?' Then there are the heavy drinking pals, who are possibly scared of facing their own issues and having you around, looking all healthy, is their worst nightmare.

So take some time to prepare. Make a list of those influential people and tackle them the old-fashioned way – in person or on the phone (see page 68).

Coming out of the alcohol closet will help in two ways. Firstly, you will make people aware of your healthy intentions, which lowers the chance of them buying you a gin and tonic by mistake. Secondly, you will be surprised at the massive support from some people and also frustrated at the reaction of others. Use the positive encouragement as extra support and the negative as motivation to prove them all wrong.

Take a few minutes and make a list of the main people you think you should speak to, using the headings here as a guide:

- **Family**
- **Friends**
- **Work colleagues.**

Now contact at least one of these people. Be firm and to the point. Refer back to all those reasons why you are taking this challenge (see page 53) and build a clear script in your mind of what you are going to say. As always, expect the unexpected. Use the 'objections' section below to prepare yourself for the counter arguments.

THE OBJECTIONS

By now we have heard every argument in the 'why you should drink' book. Here are some of the most common objections, so you can arm yourself against them:

— **Stop being so boring**
— **But drinking is fun!**
— **How are you going meet girls/boys?**
— **You need to relax**
— **It's good to have a blow-out once in a while**
— **But you have to have a drink with your old pal! You've changed.**

Write down the objections above and add some more of your own, then build a counter argument for each one. Rehearse these stories in your mind or write down your arguments. That way, when you need to defend yourself against one of these objections, you will be ready.

Hearing these objections is always slightly disappointing, but from our experience we have found that over time everyone will end up supporting you on this challenge. Those early objections will vanish once friends and family see for themselves the difference that being alcohol-free is making to your world.

WHAT IS BOOZE, REALLY …?

The Stoic philosophers prized self-discipline and worked tirelessly to master their temptations. One method they used was to strip the object of their desire back to its core elements. By scraping back the myth and mystery that surrounded their cravings, the Stoics could see each desire for what it really was and not be seduced by its story.

This is a great tool. When all the gloss is taken away, the labels are removed and social pressure is released, what's left? What is this liquid that we have all sorts of pet names for?

Ask Google 'What is alcohol' and this is what it tells you:

'A colourless volatile flammable liquid which is produced by the natural fermentation of sugars and is the intoxicating constituent of wine, beer, spirits and other drinks, and is also used as an industrial solvent and as fuel.'

Let's do a quick mind experiment to drive this alcohol-free hack home.

Imagine you are in a bar and you're handed a bottle marked with a skull and crossbones, indicating that it was poisonous. You read the label and it says, 'Contains a colourless flammable liquid that is used as an industrial solvent and as fuel.'

Would you drink it?

DAY 4

‹YOU WILL PERFORM BETTER, MAKE BETTER DECISIONS AND HAVE A BETTER BODY WHEN YOU GET THE SLEEP YOU REQUIRE›

SHAWN STEVENSON [16]

SLEEPING BEAUTY

YOUR NEW ROUTINES

You will hear us say this a lot: bad habits don't need telling off, they need replacing. This is the key finding from the science of habit-change; you keep the same trigger and reward and you simply replace an unhealthy routine with a healthy one.

 Today we want to expand on the routines section of the habit loop. The idea is to keep working on your habit loops to gain a deep understanding of this process and to bring your subconscious routines into the light of consciousness.

So, spend the next few minutes jotting down as many healthy routines as you can think of that will replace your current drinking routines.

Here are some more ideas from people just like you:

— **Swap the alcoholic beer for a non-alcoholic alternative**
— **Exercise**
— **Read**
— **Meditate**
— **Go to the cinema**
— **Go to the theatre**
— **Take a spin class**
— **Take a course to learn something new.**

The list is endless and personal to you. Freestyle your list and come up with as many

RUARI'S STORY

I came up with a couple of new routines to replace the old drinking ones. Firstly, when I realised my Friday nights at the pub was just me craving social interaction with the lads, I knew I needed to find another way. So I got a group of them together and we took up a private boxing evening. It was great fun, and the lads got some man time together. Secondly, my old routine, after a long day and once the kids were in bed, was to reward myself with wine. To replace this routine I made the extra effort to do 15 minutes of yoga using an app on my phone and 15 minutes of mindfulness. My evenings are so much calmer now and I feel better in myself. Making these small changes can have a big effect on your life in the long term.

alternative activities as possible to help you build new, healthier routines.

TAKE THE RINGLEADERS OUT OF THE EQUATION

As we suggested in Day 3, we all have those friends who are the ringleaders; you know, the guys and gals who hold court and basically take the piss out of anyone who steps out of line. They are often very witty and great fun to be around, but if they are not on board with the challenge they can seriously ramp up the pressure for you to have a drink. When faced with this overwhelming social force, best-laid intentions are often sabotaged in order to get a break from the incessant torment.

There is an old saying: 'Take out the biggest one first', and this is true in these situations. You know who these people are and how they might react. Where possible, you want to avoid a verbal battle in the bar.

On Day 3 we talked about coming out of the alcohol closet, but very often these 'ringleaders' are not the ones you initially want to approach. However, if a social event is looming and you have one of these types in your social circle, prior preparation is key.

Before you head out with the gang, meet or call the ringleader. This is not a 'text' moment. Tell them all the reasons why you're on this challenge (refer to Day 1) and combine this with counter arguments to any objections (Day 3). Make it clear how passionate you are about this challenge and

that you would like their support. Once away from the crowd, these mates are often the first to show their encouragement and can turn out to be your most powerful supporters.

This show of solidarity can make a massive difference. If you have the ringleader's seal of approval the rest of the group will often follow. Job done.

THE FIRST SOCIAL DRINK

Very early in your challenge it is likely that you will be faced with your 'first social drink'. It will be the moment when you hear those time-honoured words:

'What do you want to drink?'

We have all been there, in that moment of panic when you have to make a split-second decision whether to drink or not. If you are not prepared for this, the beer fear takes over, old habits reign supreme and you will make poor choices.

'Winging it' does not work.

The beer fear is powerful during this early stage – old habits and unhealthy routines are ready to take control. To avert this, you need to know exactly what you will say and how you will say it.

Just like athletes readying themselves for the starter's gun, you must prepare for the barman's question. Let's start our training by dipping into the worlds of sports psychology and NLP with a technique that is the secret weapon of many a world-class athlete.

VISUALISE YOUR WAY TO CHALLENGE VICTORY

Find somewhere quiet and take a couple of minutes to prepare for your first drink challenge. Close your eyes and take a few deep breaths, let yourself relax, so that you feel calm, yet alert and powerful.

Now imagine your local bar, or wherever you might face your first temptation. Try to build up a clear mental image of how it will look and what it will feel like. Use all your senses to create a vivid picture in your mind. What can you hear? What can you smell?

Once you have this picture in your mind, here comes the hard bit. Imagine yourself being asked, 'What do you want to drink?' Calmly and firmly select your healthy option. It could be a non-alcoholic beer, a soda with lime, water or juice. The key is to rehearse this in your mind until it becomes your automatic response.

'Could I have a [fill in blank], please.'

Have a variety of options in your mind. For example, you might order a NA beer only for the barman to inform you that they don't sell NA beer. By having a second or third choice in mind you prevent yourself from defaulting to the easy answer of 'Oh, erm, just a beer then.'

Run through a few scenarios in your mind until you feel confident. Five to 10 times is often enough to make a difference. It only takes a matter of seconds to perform each scenario, so feel free to keep going to really cement these healthy routines in your mind. The more effort you put in, the more you will get out of this.

Once you're confident within a particular scenario, start to mix it up and plan for different situations. Perhaps imagine various friends asking the question, 'What are you drinking?'. Or change the setting completely and visualise a nightclub or the local bar while sitting at home on the sofa. Be creative – it's your mind and your preparation. The more you practise, the better prepared you will be for the reality.

Great work! You just performed your first visualisation. We did not want to stick a label on it until you had experienced this skill for yourself. This is such a powerful technique and one that we will use many times during this challenge.

The beauty of visualisation is that you can imagine any scenario in an instant and practise, practise, practise, responding to various situations. This is why top-class athletes use visualization; they cannot physically rehearse for every given scenario on the track or the pitch, but they can walk through thousands of scenarios in their minds. They cannot physically practise their reactions to hearing the starter's gun thousands of times, but they can mentally prepare in this way. The research suggests that our minds cannot really tell the difference between a made-up scenario (visualisation) and the real thing[17]. By rehearsing healthy routines over and over, you harness the power of visualisation to reprogramme your brain and support your new healthy habits.

SLEEPING BEAUTY

During this early part of the challenge you might already feel an improvement in the quality of your sleep. On the flip side, it is around now that many members find getting to sleep difficult.

Alcohol and sleep have a troubled relationship. On the one hand, it sends us off to the sandman quickly, but once we're asleep alcohol gets up to its usual tricks and destroys the quality of our shuteye.

There is another problem – many of our members have used alcohol as a sleeping pill, so for them it is the physical act of getting to sleep that becomes an issue.

SO WHAT'S GOING ON?

In an interview with Shawn Stevenson, author of *Sleep Smarter*, on our OYNB podcast, he suggests the reason you might suffer restless nights early in the alcohol-free process is to do with how the body deals with toxicity. The liver is a beautiful protective organ that hangs on to toxins for days at a time to protect us from damage. Over the first few days of this challenge the body slowly starts to dump this metabolic waste, but this disposal takes time because the lymphatic system does not have a pump like the circulatory system has the heart. Sleep speeds up this process, but the paradox is that getting to sleep is often a problem. So Stevenson recommends two things:

First, being aware of this potential issue and taking a proactive stance rather than a reactive one can make a difference. So use all the tips listed opposite to prepare for a quality night's sleep. Make sure that you do this before bed tonight.

Secondly, the best thing you can do to help this detoxification process is to exercise. Stevenson explains that in order to help the lymphatic system clear out waste we need to move. This is another reason why exercise is key to this challenge.

Also, timing is important; when studies compared evening, afternoon and morning exercisers, it was those who were moving earliest in the day who noticed the greatest improvement in sleep-related benefits[18].

The earlier exercisers spent the most time in deep sleep, while experiencing a whopping 25 per cent greater drop in blood pressure – which turns off the fight or flight system – and in general their sleep cycles were much more efficient.

Meditation is another wonderful sleeping aid, and with a bit of effort will easily replace the booze. Check out www.oneyearnobeer.com/book-resources for some free guided audio meditations, visualisations and also some book ideas to help hack your sleeping habits.

PREPARE FOR BED

 This alcohol-free challenge provides the perfect platform to improve your sleeping habits and receive all the amazing benefits that this brings. Below are some top tips for a great night's sleep. Your mission today is to implement as many of these ideas as possible. Then, in a week's time, make a note of how much better you feel.

1. Quit the caffeine after 2p.m.

This is not just the obvious coffee; caffeine is found in many things from tea to fizzy drinks. If the labels shout 'energy', they are best avoided.

2. Avoid hot baths before bed

The body needs to be a certain temperature to be ready for sleep. Hot baths can delay this process.

3. Prepare the room

If you can, dim the lights before you go to sleep. Turn off all other lights where possible. If you like to read, use the lowest light possible and remove all bright phones that are on charge.

4. Love the dark

Our bodies are programmed to sleep when it's dark. Any light inhibits the production of the sleep hormone melatonin, because our body becomes confused between night and day. If you can, invest in proper blackout blinds or very thick curtains, as they will make a massive difference. If you can't black out the room, try a sleep mask.

5. Chill out

Your body temperature drops when sleeping, so keeping the room cooler will help with this process. Aim for 5–10 degrees Celsius lower than daytime temperatures. As always, experiment with what works for you.

6. Silent night

If you live in a noisy area, try ear plugs or even use a white-noise background soundtrack to help muffle outside disturbances.

7. Invest in an old-school alarm clock

Many of us now use our smartphones as alarm clocks. How often, when setting the alarm, have you noticed an email or text that sets your mind racing just before bed? Or you check social media or send an email right at the critical point when you should be relaxing? Also, the bright light from the phone starts to mess with your sleeping signals. So give yourself a chance and remove all phones and gadgets from the room. Aim to use an alarm clock to gently wake you after a great night's sleep.

In summary, a good night's sleep starts the moment you wake. So use all the tips above to prepare for a quality night's sleep, then exercise. This could be a jog, yoga, some loving, kettle-bell swings – or all four!

DAY 5

'I'VE MISSED MORE
THAN 9,000 SHOTS
IN MY CAREER.
I'VE LOST ALMOST
300 GAMES.
26 TIMES, I'VE BEEN
TRUSTED TO TAKE
THE GAME WINNING
SHOT AND MISSED.
I'VE FAILED OVER
AND OVER AND OVER
AGAIN IN MY LIFE.
AND THAT IS
WHY I SUCCEED'
MICHAEL JORDAN [19]

PREPARE FOR THE AMBUSH

TRIGGER HAPPY

Now you've identified some routines and rewards, let's re-examine your triggers. A key element of habit-change is spotting those moments, people, experiences or emotions that cause us to reach for a drink. The more triggers you identify, the higher the likelihood that you will notice and deal with these cravings as they happen. Once you are aware of what's driving your habits you regain so much control. From this vantage point you can enjoy the healthy routines that fulfil the reward you seek while also hacking your habit.

Take five minutes to list as many triggers as you can possibly think of. Use the five elements below to help:

— **Location**
— **Time**
— **Emotional state**
— **Other people**
— **Preceding action.**

At this stage you will have a selection of triggers and routines while you will also be beginning to understand more about the rewards you seek.

THE AMBUSH

Imagine the situation: you arrive at the bar all geared up with your challenge excuse. You enter and … wallop! One of your friends, who has yet to hear of your mission, hands you a drink.

Suddenly you're holding a beer or a glass of wine. What next?

DON'T PANIC – the beer fear will kick in, but take a deep breath, stand firm, smile and remember: YOU DON'T HAVE TO DRINK IT JUST BECAUSE SOMEONE BOUGHT IT FOR YOU!

It's only a drink, not a gold Rolex. Alcohol rarely goes to waste – someone will drink it – so don't let this be an excuse to swerve from your chosen path. Know this – you will be ambushed at some point. Then, as always, a bit of preparation will help.

Below is an example of how to respond to a classic ambush, when handed a drink:

'Sorry, I didn't get a chance to tell you, but I am on this alcohol-free challenge and I'm loving it! One of the others can have it, or save it for the next round. I'll have a non-alcoholic beer [sparkling water, fruit juice…whatever].'

At this juncture be prepared for the usual:

'Don't be a [fill in blank] – just drink it.'

Be strong.

'Sorry, I have committed to this alcohol-free challenge – the clue is in the title. I feel great and I'm determined to make it to the end.'

For extra power, cite your reasons for taking the challenge and what you want to achieve from it. Good friends will always support you.

Develop your own way of saying the same thing, but whatever it is, just like a good boy scout or girl guide, always be prepared.

There are hundreds of different scenarios that could lead you away from your goals. As on Day 3, take five minutes to note down a few and consider how you will react to each situation. Mentally rehearse what you will do and what you will say. Practise, practise, practise – in front of the mirror, in the car, on the loo – say it out loud, firm and proud:

'I am on an alcohol-free challenge and I'm loving it!'

Let's inject some reality into the alcohol/social situation. There is a tendency to believe that the majority of our social time revolves around alcohol, when this is simply not the case. While it's true that a lot of pre-planned social interactions might involve alcohol, this does not equate to your whole social life.

When you dig deeper into your social interactions you will discover that they happen all the time in a non-structured fashion. In fact, you will probably find that you already spend more time being social in your daily lives without alcohol than with it. Most of us experience great laughs, wonderful conversation and human connection nowhere near the bar. The shared joke in the office, the chat with the postman or phone call with a best mate add up to some of our best alcohol-free interactions.

Alcohol might have played a part in your social life, but let's agree that it is only a part. Most of us are already perfectly capable of having a laugh and not being boring without alcohol.

Today, take notice of all the social interactions you have that do not involve alcohol. Make a note of all the laughs and quality chats you have during the day that are a million miles from the bar. Let's start injecting a little reality back into your social world.

THE SLIP-UP

No one is perfect – Superman without kryptonite would be boring. Every now and then, one of our many perfectly human imperfections will catch us out. We eat the cake, drink the beer, smoke the cigarette and what do we do? We say to ourselves, 'What the hell, I may as well be hung for a sheep as a lamb.' This opens the floodgates, the wheels come off and so begins a massive session.

Many of us have a misguided belief that the best way to motivate ourselves is with the stick of guilt. However, it is forgiveness that helps you stay on track to achieve your goals. Researchers have found time and time again that forgiveness leads to personal accountability, whereas guilt leaves us looking for excuses[20].

Those who show self-compassion are excused from seeing themselves as losers, unlike guilt, where the shame of failure drives people to overindulge to escape these feelings. People who show self-compassion are willing to take feedback and reflect on the situation to see how they can improve.

The very idea of this experience is that you face four weeks fully alcohol-free, but if you do slip up you have a couple of options. If it was a mere blip, for example you had a sip of wine or found yourself with a bottle of beer, you can decide if this was a big enough indiscretion to start the 28 days over or carry on regardless.

The point is this: if you get to 28 days alcohol-free with only one tiny slip, that is still fantastic. We have discovered that by continuing and not letting the floodgates open, you learn so much, and if you decide to take the challenge further you might find yourself at 90 days with one blip, which would be amazing. The longer you can go without alcohol, the better. Each day is a chance to learn and reprogramme your habit systems.

What we are trying to achieve here is to give you space to help you treat yourself with compassion and nip a wobble in the bud. The science suggests that the 'What the hell effect' is waiting to kick in once you make the first mistake, when this is not helpful and offers an easy way out. So if you do trip up, just smile, learn, stop the slip-up from escalating and carry on with your challenge.

However, if you feel you want to start again, go for it. Or if one drink turned into many, dust yourself off and start from scratch. The choice, as always, is yours. But whatever you do, never, never, never give up.

IT WAS A SUCH A GREAT NIGHT

During our challenge people wanted to express their opinions about our life-changing decision to stop drinking. Some weren't able to understand why we had given up something they perceived as so enjoyable. They're not at fault; they were still enjoying alcohol – and that's completely fine.

So when someone says that drinking is fun, it is a personal opinion, nothing more. In their survey of one, they have concluded that drinking is enjoyable.

Research suggests that 83 per cent of the adult population in the UK drink alcohol[21]. This means that in the UK alone there are over 33 million drinkers, all with different views about booze. For some, it's great, while others have connected it with the experience of the breakdown of relationships, marriages and careers. Only you can decide if this pastime is fun for you, or not.

We both had enjoyed some really fun times when drinking, but rather than glorify these moments in alcohol folklore as we tend to, we decided to analyse these social occasions. We wanted to know, were we having great times because of alcohol or was it something else? So we created a simple process to check. After each social event we asked the following:

— **What was the best part of the night?**
— **When did we laugh most?**
— **When was the best conversation had?**
— **What was the worst part of the night?**
— **How did we feel the day after?**

As we answered these questions the same pattern emerged. The really fun parts of the evening came early on, when most of us were sober or merely tipsy. In this period we had the best laughs as the lads were on top form and were sharp enough to create a great atmosphere. However, as the evenings progressed and we started to get drunk, the pattern changed, or simply vanished along with our memory. When we repeated this questioning the pattern looked the same. The parts that we remembered and really enjoyed were just being with our mates and having a laugh – it was the social interaction that we craved, the booze was just an excuse for us to be together. At the same time, we exposed the parts of the evening that were pretty awful and certainly not fun:

the drunken argument, the tears and loss of function. All of these negatives appeared when drunk.

Next we looked at collateral damage and realised we were losing day after day to hangovers and regret. How could we let this self-inflicted sickness rob us of our most precious asset, time? The penny had dropped – it was our friends and the social occasion that made our evenings fun. Alcohol was not bringing the fun factor, it was there already.

We had to repeat this process a few times because we could not understand why on earth we had not worked this out before.

The trouble is, you can't kid a kidder, yet we try our best to kid ourselves all the time. How many times had we woken up the day after feeling like death, only to fabricate a story to justify the pain? If we took a survey of how many 'great nights' we had, the next morning we'd say it was close to 100 per cent. The truth is, the vast majority of drunken nights are average at best.

Some of you reading this might not agree. Only a few years ago WE wouldn't have agreed either. However, as Ruari has now learnt, although sometimes it helps to grease the wheels, the moment this becomes a regular thing, the whole plan can start to break down.

For every fantastic evening there are always a few that don't end that well. That's why taking an extended break is so important because your true perspective returns and you see alcohol for what it is.

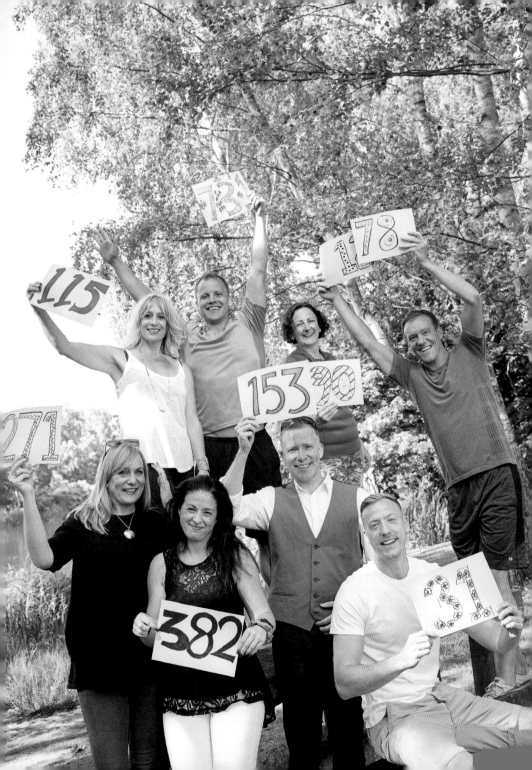

DAY 6

'IT SHOULD BE COOL TO GIVE. IT SHOULD BE COOL TO BE GENEROUS. IT SHOULD BE COOL TO SAY YES TO HELPING OUT'
SCOTT HARRISON [22]

ALWAYS HAVE A BACKUP PLAN

THE PULL OF A PINT

At this stage you are familiar with your triggers and have some healthy routines. Now let's take a closer look at the rewards you crave.

The next time you feel a craving for a drink, perform the following exercise:

STEP 1

When you feel a craving coming on, play one of your selected healthy routines. Then take a quick break and note down the first three things that come to mind. Don't worry what the words are, they can be meaningless; the important thing is to note them down. The reason we want you make a note of these words is because in doing so we are forcing you to think about your actions, rather than allowing yourself to work on autopilot. Also these words will later help jog your memory about how you felt at that particular moment.

STEP 2

Now set your alarm for 15 minutes' time and note down how you feel once again. Has the craving gone? Do you feel satisfied? Has the reward you were seeking been fulfilled by the healthy routine you played? If so, you know that this is the perfect routine for your reward.

For example, if you guessed that your reward was the ability to relax after a long day at work and you replaced the glass of wine with a long hot bath or some 'me' time to read a book, then after 15 minutes you felt relaxed and the craving had gone – you were right. Relaxation was the reward you were after and now you have a fantastic healthy routine to play instead.

Perhaps you guessed that your reward was to feel the social bonds of being with a group and you replaced the drinks after work with a bike ride with your friends, but then 15 minutes after the ride you still felt something was missing, so it might not have been the social aspect you craved. In this example you might take another guess at what your reward might be. Perhaps it was to let off some steam about your annoying boss. In this example you could keep the drinks after work as your reward to let off some steam and replace the alcohol routine with an alcohol-free alternative. Once again, check 15 minutes after the activity to see if it fulfilled your desired reward.

The aim here is to help you identify the reward that is driving this habit. Keep experimenting with these ideas until you create several healthy routines for the rewards you commonly crave, such as relaxation, stress relief, social contact and so on. The more you learn about your inner world the more capable of positive change you will become.

☑ HAVE A BACKUP PLAN A, B, C, D …

Having spent many evenings out searching for non-alcoholic beer, we have discovered that it's not well-stocked. Bars are better than restaurants, but many establishments don't offer a non-alcoholic 'lookalike' option. Therefore, if you intend to start with non-alcoholic alternatives, have a backup plan. We have all been undone by this basic error of judgement. We have walked into the bar full of good intentions, only to reach the counter, order a non-alcoholic option and discover there is none. Old habits take over, and before we know it, the beer fear kicks in and we make the wrong choice.

This is where your soft-drink backup plan comes into action. If plan A is not an option, have a plan B. Order a sparkling water and add a mixer straw and a slice of lemon. It's a dead ringer for a gin and tonic. It's these small victories that will help you on this challenge. All too often it's the little things that trip us up. Prepare, prepare, prepare.

I DESERVE A DRINK

After a stressful week or day, how many times have you uttered the words, 'I deserve a drink'?

As we started to analyse our worlds we noticed that we often rewarded good behaviour with the very thing we were avoiding. A week off the booze was rewarded with a beer. We wondered why had we built a reward system that was the polar opposite of the activity we were being rewarded for?

MORAL LICENSING

Psychologists call this type of thinking moral licensing[23], and its effects have been proven in the lab time and time again. Research has demonstrated that if dieters are reminded of how well they're doing and are then offered an apple or chocolate, a staggering 85 per cent take the chocolate. This works both ways. When participants were asked to remember a time when they acted generously, right before they made a charitable donation, they went on to donate 60 per cent less than those who were not asked this question.

This moral licensing allows us to do things that are opposed to our goals, buying us credits to make dubious choices today that are based on past acts of virtue. Not drinking alcohol for a week allows us to reward ourselves with the very thing we have been avoiding – a drink.

It's the same with exercise; some people will work their socks off all week to stay in shape and then reward themselves with pizza at the weekend.

Moral licensing occurs when we label things as good and bad. Not drinking alcohol = good, drinking alcohol = bad. Staying alcohol-free is mentally building up lots of 'good' points, and what do points make? Prizes! Tonight's special prize is a beer.

In order to remove this imaginary points system, 'I deserve a drink' had to be replaced with something new that was in keeping with our healthy alcohol-free mission. Remember, you cannot win today's game with yesterday's points!

After studying our own reward systems, we decided that with a little effort we could put some new ones in place. We would replace the beer with a take-away of our choice. Ok, it's not necessarily the healthiest reward, but it was a step in the right direction and the challenge means little steps. Thus 'I deserve a drink' became 'I deserve a take-away.' Over time we phased out the take-away and replaced it with healthy options such as a run, a trip to the theatre or a total chill on the sofa. But to kick it off we kept it nice and simple – a take-away replaced beer.

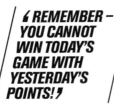

❛ REMEMBER – YOU CANNOT WIN TODAY'S GAME WITH YESTERDAY'S POINTS!❜

THREE FOODS WITH AS MANY HEALTH BENEFITS AS RED WINE

If the heart-health benefit of red wine was your main 'excuse' to drink it, try these antioxidant-rich foods instead:

— **Red and black grapes**
— **All sorts of berries**
— **A couple of squares of high-quality very dark chocolate.**

CHANGE YOUR REWARD SYSTEMS

Today, make some time to evaluate your reward systems. How could you treat yourself for having completed a full week alcohol-free?

Conjure up as many ideas as you can. There are no wrong or right answers here. Perhaps you could use some of the extra cash you have saved to treat yourself. Put these rewards in place so that your good points create a 'good' reward that fits in with your new healthy goals.

You don't have to apply this only to your alcohol-free challenge, you could put some healthy rewards in place for a week's worth of exercise or study, too.

GOOD REWARD BOOSTER

 Let's use a simple visualisation technique to prepare for when the wrong reward comes knocking.

Start by taking a few deep breaths. When you feel ready, close your eyes and feel yourself relaxing with each out breath.

Imagine feeling great for amassing lots of 'good' points, then suddenly you're tempted by the wrong reward. Now instead of eating cake or drinking the beer, replace this reward in your mind with one of the alternative rewards you just created.

Imagine how natural it feels to make the right choice, to be rewarded with something that does not conflict with your goals. Bathe in the warm feelings that this creates. Do you feel good about yourself? Do you feel content for a job well done? Enjoy this process of receiving the right reward. Well done, you deserve it.

Perform this visualisation using various scenarios that might tempt you. Each time, imagine that you respond the right way by selecting a reward that is in keeping with your long-term goals.

Perform this exercise as many times as you feel is necessary to train your mind to react in the right fashion. Between five and 10 times is often enough.

CHARITY MATE

We know all about the social pressure that engulfs alcohol. Well, here is a clever hack that pays out a double win and turns this social pressure on its head. Why not take this challenge for charity?

The benefits are two-fold. Firstly, you will raise money for those in need, which is a beautiful thing. Secondly, you can leverage the same social pressure that wants to keep you drinking to keep you ... from drinking. Making a commitment to charity will build social pressure in the right way. You will not want to let down either the charity or those people who sponsor you. This healthy pressure will keep you on the right track during the early weeks.

Be loud and proud; you are not only changing your life for the better, you are trying to help others. What an amazing goal – and something that we would wager most of your friends and family will support.

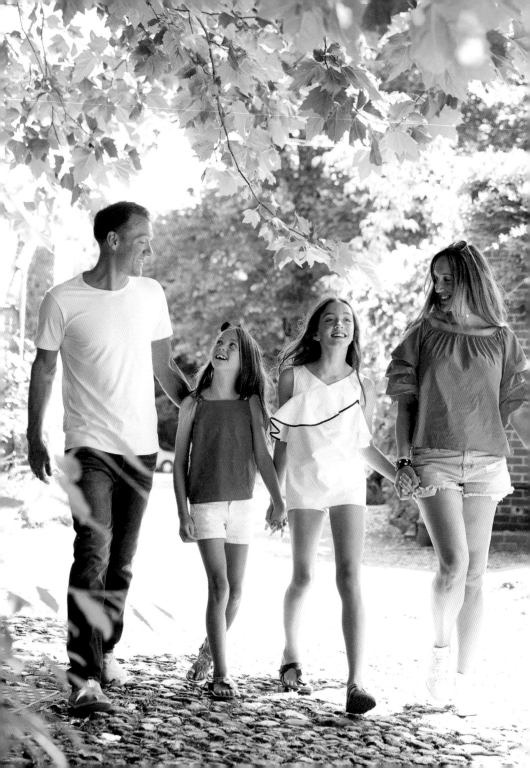

DAY 7

‹THERE ARE BETTER STARTERS THAN ME BUT I'M A STRONG FINISHER›

USAIN BOLT [24]

FIND A GOAL FRIEND

HACK YOUR SOCIAL LIFE

Here's an idea – rather than swapping alcohol for alcohol-free during your social events, why not do something totally different?

☑ If your current social life usually revolves around booze, mix things up a little. Perhaps arrange a bowling night or try go-karting. Meet the gang for a day out mountain biking or hiking. It takes a little effort to think of something to do, but these alternative social events often beat the overdone drinking session hands down. Those alcohol-loving friends will happily plod along with the same old same old until someone – you – shakes things up.

The beauty of the alcohol-free activity is that friends appreciate the effort. While another drinking session blurs into all the others, a night go-karting or a city ghost tour can make a lasting impression. Also, because you are at the cutting edge of a major paradigm shift in attitudes towards alcohol, friends will love to feel that they were part of something ahead of time.

The extra bonus is that by removing the alcohol you are back on a level playing field and temptation is a million miles away. You can be a social butterfly without worrying about the alcohol situation.

THE HABIT 100M

💡 Professional athletes all over the land use visualisation to prepare for races, but these skills are not just reserved for the elite few. As you discovered on Day 4, you can apply this technique to create powerful healthy habits.

TRY THIS EXERCISE:

Look at your list of triggers and healthy routines, then note down a few combinations that you might encounter. For example:

Trigger
6 p.m. need to de-stress.
Routine
Talk a walk outside in nature.

Trigger
Stressful day at work.
Routine
Listen to some of your favourite tunes.

Once you have a few combinations in mind, take a few minutes to perform the following exercise.

Start with a few deep breaths. When you feel ready, close your eyes and feel yourself relaxing with each exhale.

Once you feel ready, imagine one of your triggers – it could be the smell of beer, the end of work or sitting on the couch after a long day. Build this trigger in your mind. Bring all your senses into play: what can you hear, taste, smell and feel? Then let the craving intensify until the trigger is fired, and now imagine that you play a new healthy routine instead of reaching for a drink.

Make this scenario bright in your mind; notice how great it feels to be doing something constructive that does not involve alcohol. What can you see, what can you sense? Notice how powerful this feels and the confidence this brings. Keep building on these feelings for a few more seconds, and if you're enjoying this process, stay with it. There are no wrong or right emotions here. Once you have played through this scenario in your mind and the healthy routine is finished, repeat the exercise a few times to drive this new habit home.

Practise with each trigger/routine combination several times, making sure these new loops set themselves in your mind.

This mental preparation will allow you to perform your reaction and rehearse your healthy habit loops over and over in your mind. When the real-life trigger occurs you will instinctively fire the new routine without thinking and hack your habit.

YOU'RE NOT FINISHED YET

Now that you're discovering how to build new healthy habits, don't be fooled into thinking you are done and dusted. You still have to plan and watch out for those unexpected moments that will test your newfound resolve. But if something does catch you out and you slip up, take comfort in the fact that you noticed. This is because your awareness is expanding and you can spot previously unconscious errors of judgement.

As always, dust yourself off, make a note of this curve ball and come back stronger. Perform your visualisations again and include the new scenario that tripped you up. This mental rehearsal will give you the strength to deal with each and every scenario. Well done.

 FIND YOURSELF A GOAL FRIEND
Take a look around. Who else might want to join you on this challenge? You'll be amazed at how many people will be inspired by your actions and the changes you're making.

Finding a non-drinking buddy can make it much easier for both of you to succeed. You can trade ideas, team up on activities and support each other socially.

Your 'goal friend' does not have to be specific or limited to this alcohol-free challenge. Look to apply the power of goal friends to all of your challenges. If you have set yourself the goal of completing a mud race, why not get your mates on board? Or if your dream is to run a marathon, find a goal friend to train with.

As always, have a look around, get creative and see if you can find a goal friend today.

Some people just won't get it ... at the moment. Your challenge will inspire many and annoy some – who will most likely be secretly inspired! Be prepared for the odd under-reaction to your challenge. These people are scared. They are scared to question their own habits because they are frightened of what they might find. Don't let these types upset you; rather you should feel empathy for them. Use these negatives to make you even more determined to succeed. The best comeback of all is action. Stay with the challenge and we wager that the very same person who right now does not understand will approach you at some point and say, 'Wow. How did you do it? I think it's time I tried.'

It's good to remember that every single one of us interprets the world and what's happening around us in a slightly different way. Put simply, we are in charge of our own reality. What we see, hear and taste is filtered through our mind, which creates emotions, feelings and reactions. It's these filters that are unique to us, formed over time from past experiences, personal beliefs and hand-me-down beliefs from influential people in our lives, such as parents and friends.

Try to imagine an infinite number of cameras all taking a picture of an object from a slightly different angle. Each photograph would be unique in angle, light and structure. It's the same when each person encounters food, drink, exercise and general day-to-day living. We all have a slightly different experience because we filter the situation through our minds.

There are two major lessons to be derived from this understanding. First, by changing the way we interpret situations, and therefore our beliefs, we can manipulate the way we feel. So rather than being dragged around by our inbuilt preconceptions, which are often misplaced, we can take back control and change our beliefs. We will show you how to do this on Day 15. Second, everyone sees the world differently, so your interpretation of how to behave can be very different from someone else's.

WHOSE INTERPRETATION IS CORRECT?

Both are correct according to each individual's filters of the situation. Therefore we have to learn tolerance of others, because our view of the world is just that, our opinion – nothing more.

Stay strong when faced with negative reactions, as it is just their view of the world at the moment. Complete the challenge and see if their view changes. Take pride in leading by example; there's no need to preach, just be the happy healthy you.

WEEK 1 – REFLECTION

WHAT ARE YOU PROUD OF?

Rather than dwell on the tough parts of this challenge, let's feed the positive vibe and list all the things you are proud of so far. These items on the list don't have to be earth-shattering; your list could include people you have met, your personal achievements or your discoveries throughout the challenge so far.

Take five minutes now to conjure up these thoughts and note them down.

Well done, you are flying into Week 2.

FILL OUT THE QUICK PROGRESS TRACKER BELOW

Give yourself a rating out of 10 for each of the categories, with 1 being a poor rating and 10 being amazing.

Better yet, record your responses so you can track your changes over time at **members.oneyearnobeer.com/Test/Week1**

QUICK PROGRESS TRACKER	
HAPPINESS	/10
MOTIVATION	/10
PRODUCTIVITY	/10
SLEEP	/10
ENERGY	/10
TIME	/10
EXERCISE	/10
OVERALL SCORE	/70

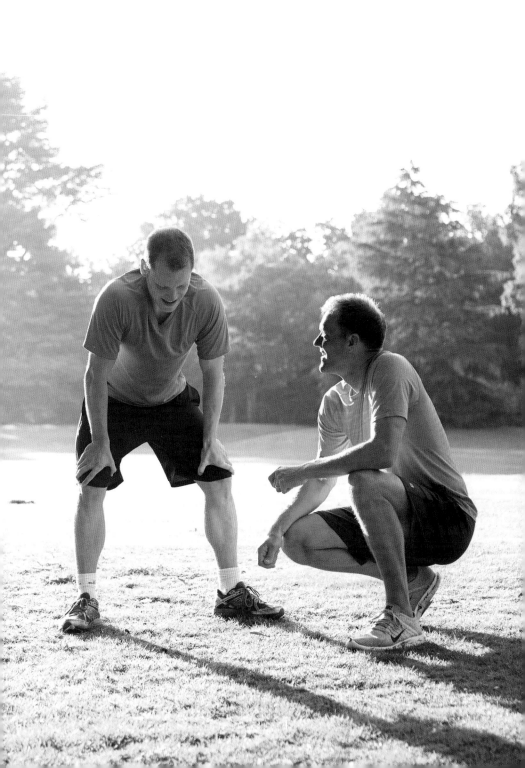

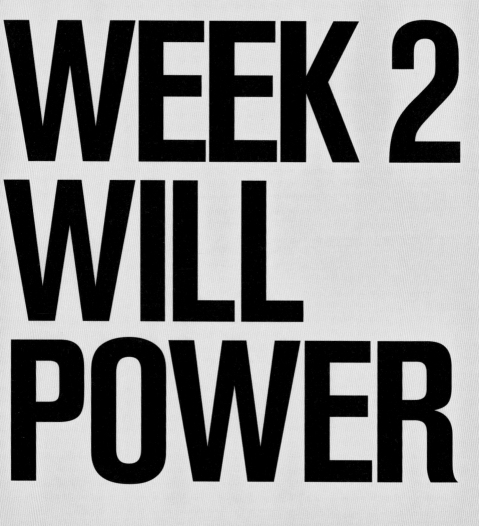

You super star, you're really hitting your stride. The alcohol is now long gone and you understand all about triggers and rewards, so now it's time to lift the lid on the often misunderstood concept of willpower. You will discover that willpower is not something you're blessed with, it's like a muscle that you can strengthen. The science, techniques and skills you will learn are all designed to pump your willpower muscles and help you take on this challenge in style.

Week 2 is often the time to move back into your normal social life, but these alcohol-free social occasions may well require an extra level of preparation so that you can enjoy them. As we progress you will uncover how to maximise your nights out and learn from a behavioural economist why it might be better to leave the party a little earlier rather than stay to the end.

It is also during this week that you might start to feel good, almost too good, and this is when people forget why they are here and slip up. So as a quick reminder, go back to all your reasons that you noted on Day 1 as to why you started out on this alcohol-free adventure. Another top tip for this week is to have a nice treat lined up to celebrate having completed two weeks booze-free. So book something exciting that will help you get over the second-week hump. Perhaps arrange to go to the theatre, a sporting match or spend time with loved ones. This reward will keep you focused and busy towards the end of the week, helping you flow nicely into Week 3.

DAY 8

‘THEY'RE TINY
THINGS BUT
IF YOU CLUMP
THEM TOGETHER
IT MAKES A BIG
DIFFERENCE’
SIR DAVID BRAILSFORD [25]

WILLPOWER PERFECTIONISTS

When everything is running smoothly this challenge can feel easy. The problem is, life does not run smoothly for long and soon the slip-up gremlins will be out in force. A maxim to remember is that we are all willpower perfectionists until we need it most. When anger starts to surface and the red mist clouds your mind, all those hours of meditation or other calming exercises seem to evaporate and emotions rule. This leads to frustration that all your effort is wasted.

It's the same with alcohol: now that your skills are growing and you have a week under your belt, you may be feeling that you have got this. Then you find yourself in a situation that you were not prepared for and a slip-up occurs. Once again, frustration reigns supreme and you are left wondering, 'Where were my alcohol-free powers when I needed them most?'

Many of us have been there – the non-alcoholic lager becomes a beer, the salad becomes a burger, the fruit becomes a cake. This is known as bounded rationality[26]. In theory, we have things under perfect control until we are faced with the real threat. At this point our primitive self takes over and we are blinded by desire. Rational decisions are temporarily suspended, and both body and mind become slave to a different master. You will find this happening many times, but take strength; this is natural and you have to train yourself to combat this cognitive blindness.

Simply becoming aware of this syndrome will help. So if your non-alcoholic option becomes a beer, remember, you don't have to drink it just because you bought it. Put the beer down, with your hands where you can see them, and move away from the alcohol. Take a deep breath, smile and re-order what you really want – a drink that fits with your long-term goals and healthy life. So you lost the money on the drink, who cares? In the long run you will be saving tons by not drinking. Stay strong, have a little chuckle and move on.

SMALL VICTORIES

Researchers have found that changing one habit can cause positive ripples throughout your life[27]. Exercising as little as once a week can spark healthy improvements without you even noticing. You drink less coffee, eat healthier food, smoke fewer cigarettes, are less stressed and tend to be more productive at work.

There is extensive research that confirms the power of these small wins. As you accomplish each little task, the likelihood of achieving your next target increases. This then snowballs, giving you more and more wins, leading to more confidence that massive change is possible. Genius!

It just so happens that taking a break from alcohol is a keystone habit that has the potential to unlock so many other well-being benefits. Now that you are a little way into your challenge, start to broaden this well-being brush and note down all those extra challenges that you could take on. Dream big and let your mind run free. You will be amazed at what you can achieve once you know how.

Why not:

— **Start a daily exercise routine or enhance an existing one?**
— **Improve or change your diet to eat like an athlete?**
— **Create a mindfulness routine and work on your mental toughness?**

Take 10 minutes to note down all those extra willpower challenges you could start today. Then look at your top three ideas and act on one of them now. Send the email, arrange the class or join the group, but make sure to action this idea – today.

MYTHBUSTER – BUT I HAVE NO WILLPOWER

One particular myth that stops people in their alcohol-free tracks is the belief that they have no willpower. We found ourselves in the same position; too many times our good intentions ended up turning from water into wine. As these moments piled up we began to doubt ourselves, concerned that we were somehow different. Perhaps we were born with zero willpower, or had picked up a disease or our genes were faulty.

This dangerous myth needs smashing. Willpower is not something that you either have or you don't have. It is like a muscle that you can build over time. For this reason many of our members end up creating exercise routines, improve their diets, lose weight, get fit, start meditating and chase their dreams.

RUARI'S STORY

When I started my I'm well known for my Haribos-eating skills; hand me the bag and they're destroyed in nanoseconds. So I bought a bag of Haribos and put them out, one by one, on top of my keyboard. This would mean that I had to stare at them during the day. I then set the timer on my phone to 15 minutes. Every 15 minutes my alarm went off with the words, 'You have a choice.' I then decided whether I wanted one or not. It was so simple, and probably a strong reason behind the success of my first year alcohol-free. This small willpower victory was a behemoth in habit-change.

Armed with this knowledge, we started to smash the willpower myth. When we tripped up, instead of being disappointed at ourselves, we looked for ways to learn how to avoid this happening again. Were we tired or hungry, or had our willpower reserves been depleted by a stressful day at work?

We started to think like athletes preparing for a race. What skills, techniques and planning would be required to stay alcohol-free? How could we reduce stress so that we could keep our willpower reserves high, what foods would nourish our bodies and minds, how could we protect our sleep? What exercises could we perform to help reprogramme our operating system to hardcode our new healthy habits?

The brain is so malleable that this extra preparation led to fewer slip-ups and longer alcohol-free streaks, which eventually led to the ultimate realisation that there is nothing to give up and everything to gain.

GO PUBLIC

Reminder: this is a challenge and nothing more – there's no stigma or labels. It is a challenge just like the thousands of others that people enjoy, from learning a new language to taking part in triathlons. Be proud of what you aim to achieve. It takes real courage to take on a social challenge such as this. We fully appreciate that not everyone will be comfortable going public, and that's fine – as always, you have to do what's right for you.

SOCIAL ANIMALS

You have already discovered how powerful the social pressure to drink is; now let's see what happens when you pile on the pressure to quit. The more people who know about your challenge, the more your pride instinct will kick in. Tell your drinking buddies, announce what you're doing on Facebook, tweet about it and sing it from the rooftops. In doing so you will unleash a whole load of social pressure behind your cause. You won't want to let some people down and you will want to prove others wrong. This is a genius way to generate bundles of extra motivation.

We have created a library of posts and images for you to share on social media that will really help you boost your success in this challenge. Check out www.oneyearnobeer.com/book-resources.

MYTHBUSTER –
ALCOHOL MAKES ME CONFIDENT

Don't get us wrong, we used to love a bit of Dutch courage; so much so that no social occasion was the same without it. The lunch meeting, the meeting with friends, the meeting about a meeting; wherever possible, any occasion that required an extra dose of confidence was fuelled by it.

If we're honest, Dutch courage has caused a lot of upset over the years. We have said and done things we deeply regret because of it: there have been fights, arguments, stupid statements, upset and a misguided notion of invincibility. It all leads to self-loathing and deep regret. Real confidence killers. So we had to face up to it: while we were drinking, we were living a lie.

Let's make this simple – alcohol did not provide any actual confidence, it just numbed our natural emotions and tricked us into believing that it did. On so many occasions we put the world to rights, told the boss where to go, started the new business, changed our life while drinking in the pub, only to see this false bravado flushed down the toilet with last night's kebab. On waking full of hangover the next day this false confidence was replaced with anxiety, fear and a total lack of confidence.

Guess what? The next time we needed some 'confidence' it was time to reach for a beer and repeat this crazy merry-go-round.

GET COMFORTABLE FEELING UNCOMFORTABLE

The skills you're learning during this challenge will help you maximise life alcohol-free, but they cannot make all your social occasions feel exactly the same as before. We cannot deny that alcohol does offer the power to reduce social worries. For example, you may have used alcohol as a social crutch to negate any anxieties by bulldozing your emotions.

So now you are back in the social mix without this crutch and you might find that you are a little uncomfortable. This is only natural and it will take a while to get used to. In fact, you might always feel somewhat uncomfortable in certain social occasions. But this is great, because this is the real you showing up. Take great comfort in the fact that this is your authentic self rather than a fake version brought on by alcohol. There is nothing wrong with feeling this way, most everyone does. You are not alone.

ANDY'S STORY

When I first went public with my challenge, two things happened. On the one hand there was real support, which was fantastic. On the other hand there were the naysayers, those who thought they knew me better. One particular 'friend' laughed and bet 'any money' that I would not last two weeks, let alone a year. This really annoyed me and, ironically, provided more motivation than all the kind-hearted support put together. So by going public you might attract positive and negative support. If you frame their power in the right way, both types can provide you with powerful motivation to change.

When we interviewed Ryan Holiday, author of *The Obstacle is the Way,* on our podcast, he remarked that he enjoyed feeling a little uncomfortable socially without alcohol. These emotions are a sign that you're uncovering who you really are.

So your social life might change and you might feel differently, but enjoy the ride, as this is an indication that you are making real progress.

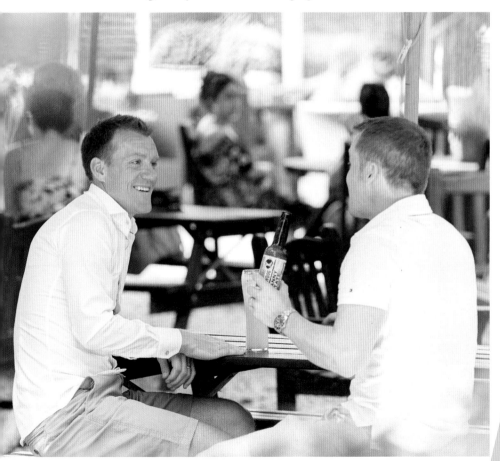

DAY 9

'DON'T USE SCEPTICISM AS A THINLY VEILED EXCUSE FOR INACTION OR REMAINING IN YOUR COMFORT ZONE'
TIM FERRIS [28]

EAT RIGHT AND HACK YOUR HABITS

We are what we eat and drink – it's as simple as that. At best, alcohol provides empty calories, while at worst (at the really heavy drinking end of things), it can lead to such an unbalanced diet that we miss out on vital nutrients. In some cases, alcohol can complicate things by also impairing the body's absorption, metabolism and utilisation of nutrients and cause malnourishment as a result – for example, of vitamins A and E.

The ideal scenario is that your alcohol-free adventure will kick-start a healthier diet. As your challenge progresses, we want you to discover ways to eat well and enjoy food without feeling you are missing out, and without substituting alcohol with another vice such as excess sugar.

Nutrition is a big topic that we can't cover in its entirety here, so our target is to provide tips that will support you in staying free from alcohol and dealing with any cravings. Eating the right types of foods at the right times will make your alcohol-free adventure easier while also improving your general health and energy levels. Stick to minimally processed 'whole' foods and you can't go far wrong.

WHAT CAN I DO TO REDRESS THE BALANCE AND FIGHT CRAVINGS?

Build your meals around adequate protein, minimally processed high-fibre carbohydrates and a ton of colourful vegetables. Make sure you throw in some healthy fats (nuts, seeds, avocados and olive oil), plus oily fish (a great source of omega 3s) in your diet at least once a week. In a strange but true twist, a pint of premium lager can contain a third of your recommended daily intake of folic acid (important for the immune system and making red blood cells), which is similar to the amount in a serving of steamed broccoli. So when you omit alcohol, be sure to eat up your greens or other good sources of folic acid, such as baked beans and potatoes.

GET A GOOD START TO THE DAY

How you start the day sets the stage for the rest of the day. A good breakfast is sensible; without it you might turn to sugary foods like biscuits or pastries mid-morning, which can set up a vicious cycle of cravings and undulating blood sugar and energy levels. Healthy breakfasts include eggs and wholegrain toast, porridge, yogurt and fruit.

PROTEIN WITH EVERY MEAL

Aim to include some source of protein – animal or vegetable – with every meal. Protein is the most satiating nutrient and can help to stabilise blood sugar levels and in turn potentially offset cravings.

This does not have to mean steak for breakfast; you could include a tablespoon of almonds or pumpkin seeds or a dairy serving with your meal, or use vegetarian proteins such as beans or tofu. Indeed, porridge made with milk has the same amount of protein as a couple of scrambled eggs.

HEALTHY CARBS

It's fashionable to cut carbohydrates, but they aren't the enemy and it's not a good idea to slash them when you're cutting out alcohol. Carbs are the body's primary source of energy and without them blood sugar can become unstable, with a knock-on effect on serotonin, a brain chemical that facilitates a stable mood. Low levels of serotonin can result in sleep problems, irritability and depression – which might encourage you to drink.

Choose healthier high-fibre sources of carbohydrates; these release more slowly and are naturally richer in nutrients – think wholemeal bread, brown rice, wholewheat pasta, quinoa, chickpeas, baked beans and other pulses and you're on the right track. (Potatoes are fine, but are better if they are cooked in their skins and are especially good when chilled in a salad.) It's the faster-releasing carbohydrates found in sugary

> *THE KEY TO ANY HEALTHY DIET: STICK WITH MINIMALLY PROCESSED "WHOLE" FOODS AND YOU CAN'T GO TOO FAR WRONG.*

foods and those with a high load of 'refined' starches (white bread, white rice and puffy savoury snacks) that are the ones to restrict.

A good rule of thumb is that half your plate should be made up of vegetables and fruit, a quarter with protein and another quarter with starchy carbohydrates.

GOOD FATS

Good fats provide the raw material for making hormone-like substances that control inflammation levels in the body (too much inflammation is linked with many aspects of ill health). Good fats are found in oily fish, avocados, all types of nuts and seeds and all kinds of olive and vegetable oils. It's a good idea to mix up lots of different types, but to ensure you get enough of the specific type of omega 3 fats that keep your heart healthy (and have the biggest anti-inflammatory effect), eat at least one portion of oily fish, such as salmon, sardines or mackerel, every week.

LOOK AFTER YOUR GUT

The trillions of bacteria in our gut (collectively known as our gut microbiome) influence many areas of health, including the immune system, and our ability to control our weight. In his book *The Diet Myth*, Tim Spector, lead investigator of the British Gut project, explains that our microbes are not only essential for digesting food, but also control the calories we absorb. If you've been a heavy drinker your gut microbiome may be sub-optimal, and a diet with lots of low-fibre processed foods will deplete the 'good' bugs in your gut bacteria, too. Studies show that the more diverse your diet, the more diverse your microbes and the better your health, at any age. Returning your gut to optimal health requires eating a wide variety of foods, especially high-fibre plant foods such as onions, leeks, garlic, and wholegrains, along with fermented foods such as yogurt and kefir.

DRINK WATER

Mild dehydration can increase food cravings, so drink regularly. The Eatwell Guide[29], which gives government recommendations on healthy eating and a balanced diet, says we should consume six to eight glasses of fluid a day – water, low-fat milk and sugar-free drinks including tea and coffee all count. How much you need depends on the weather conditions and how active you are. The best guide is to check your urine; a pale straw colour means you are drinking the right amount.

SURF THE URGE

The surfing the urge meditation is not just reserved for alcohol craving, you can apply the exact same technique to overcome any sort of temptation (see page 158).

FOCUS ON SWEET EXPERIENCES, NOT ALCOHOL AND SWEET FOOD

Experiences, interactions, social connections, awe and bliss. Seek out and savour the positive moments in your life. Make an effort to create pleasure and enjoyment in watching a sunset, a live theatre performance, having an uplifting conversation with a good friend or engaging in a fun hobby.

MAGNESIUM

One of the minerals we are most likely to not get enough of is magnesium. Taking supplements (the Recommended Daily Allowance is 375mg) may help if you often feel tired, stressed and have fluctuating energy levels. One of the effects of magnesium – along with chromium – is to help the body respond to sugar better.

THE SUGAR MONSTER

Anecdotally, sweet cravings may be more of a problem when you first stop drinking. On one level it's ok to replace an alcoholic beverage with another treat (you could argue that you've earned the calories, after all), but it's not a great idea in the long term. You can, of course, enjoy food that you love – no diet is sustainable if you don't – but don't just substitute one unhealthy pleasure for another. Dried and fresh fruit may prevent you reaching for cake, chocolate or biscuits.

DAY 10

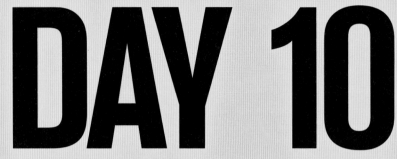

‘IF YOU DON'T LOOK AFTER YOUR BODY YOU WILL HAVE NOWHERE TO LIVE’

JASON VALE [30]

THE FIRST BIG SOCIAL EVENT

At some point during your challenge you will face a big social event – it could be a wedding, work drinks, a college reunion, a birthday or just a party. If this happens very early in your challenge, don't try to be a willpower super hero, just make time to plan ahead. There is an argument that these events are best avoided early on in the challenge, but in many ways meeting them full on is a great way to learn and experience makes all subsequent events easier to handle.

We totally understand that one of the toughest parts of this challenge is overcoming the big social occasion, but doing so is one of the most rewarding and motivational parts of this challenge. Whether you're a social drinker or you prefer to drink at home, when the big event comes knocking we are all in the same position. It is often these moments that we fear the most, but just imagine how cool it will be to take on the big event in alcohol-free style. Wouldn't it be great to turn up to that wedding and have an amazing time, alcohol-free?

The great news is, you can! Over time we learned that if we prepared ourselves in advance we could breeze through these social events. They were a little different to how they had been before, but they were actually even more enjoyable with a clear head. Also, the confidence we gained by thriving during these events helped propel us towards challenge success. Once you have enjoyed a wedding alcohol-free, a night out with a few friends is easy.

So our advice is to take it easy during the early days. Don't try to be hero if you can avoid it, but if you're called into social action, prepare for it like an alcohol-free athlete.

BREAK GLASS IN CASE OF EMERGENCY

It is impossible for us to predict when your big event might arise and what type of occasion it could be. So before your big event, head to the 'Break glass in case of Emergency' section (page 208) where we have compiled a list of the best tips and tricks to smash any social occasion from holidays to stag/hen parties.

WILLPOWER IS A FINITE RESOURCE

As we've said already, willpower is like a muscle that you can strengthen, and in more ways than one.

If you have spent the day resisting the temptation to scream at your boss, by the time your spin class comes around your willpower resources will be depleted. Too often you skip the class and miss the chance to exercise. If your day is stressful, your willpower muscles will be working hard to prevent you losing the plot, so any willpower challenge you face in the evening will be harder than anything you have faced in the morning when the same muscles are rested. This explains why many of us find it easier to exercise in the mornings, when our willpower tanks are full.

 ## PUMP THOSE WILLPOWER MUSCLES

This challenge is about pumping up those willpower muscles to help you create more healthy habits and routines. Depending on your lifestyle, these muscles will tire, so plan your willpower challenges for when your energy stores are full.

For example, if you feel your willpower is tested daily and you want to create a weekly exercise routine, plan to exercise before the day gets underway. If mornings are not an option, you will require extra motivation to make those evening sessions, so perhaps pre-arrange to meet a friend who you won't want to let down.

You get the idea – if your willpower reserves could be low, conjure up ideas to give them a boost to help you stay on track with your chosen goals.

In these early days, try to avoid or move any social occasions that might follow a stressful day when your willpower reserves might be low. If you do have to attend, make some time to de-stress before you go. Exercise or meditation might help. Over time you will know when your reserves are full, when they need a little top-up, and what works for you.

LET'S GET MOVING

A recent study by Public Health England[31] reported that eight out of 10 adults between the ages of 40 and 60 were living unhealthy lives. This is crazy when we know what we should eat and why we should exercise daily. We also know that we should drink less. So why is this happening, why are these stats so awful? Clearly it's not a lack of knowledge, but a lack of action that's the problem. That's why this challenge is perfect, because it helps you to make things happen.

There are hundreds of ways to get fit without having to hit the gym. Experiment with your world and try hobbies that get you moving. Could you join a club or arrange to go for a jog with friends? Perhaps think outside the box and look at different sports such as table tennis, orienteering or foot golf? The options are limitless. If you can't think of anything just now, put on your trainers and go for a walk. Take action and make this happen today.

JOIN YOUR LOCAL PARKRUN

Parkruns are timed, 5k, free events that take place on Saturdays at 9a.m. all over the world. You can walk, jog, run, bring the dog or the kids in a pram. So there is no excuse and almost everyone can take part. This is such a fantastic way to exercise and meet new people.

Right now, head over to parkrun.com to find your local Parkrun. There is bound to be one near you. All you have to do is sign up and go!

HEALTH BY STEALTH

Let's aim to create exercise where previously only the mundane existed. A ton of exercise opportunities often goes unnoticed throughout the day. A great example is the commute to work. Could you jump off the train two stops early and jog or walk the rest of the way? Or could you park the car a few kilometres from your workplace and run the last stretch? What about simply using the stairs rather than the lift, or getting a standing desk? Perhaps you could purchase a bike and cycle in. You get the idea; with a little planning you could build stealth exercise that also gets you from A to B as part of your normal day.

Take a few minutes now to think about your day and see where you could create some stealth exercise.

Note down at least two stealth exercise ideas. Get creative with your world. Put at least one of these ideas in place today and make it happen!

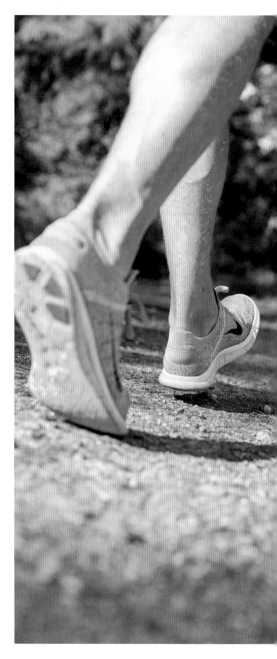

DO A HIIT (HIGH INTENSITY INTERVAL TRAINING) WORKOUT

These short, sharp workouts can make a real difference. You only need 20 minutes, three times a week and no equipment is required, so you can perform these sessions anywhere – they are effective and get results. This short-burst exercise programme brings down your levels of cortisol (stress hormone) and insulin (fat-storing hormone). When those hormones are reduced, hunger and cravings come down as well. A win–win.

Here is a basic HIIT workout for you to try:

Warm up

Always make sure you warm up before you start any exercise.

Jog or march on the spot for 30 seconds.

Stand tall and circle your arms backwards, as if you were swimming backstroke, for 30 seconds.

Finally, perform one minute of air squats – move your body down into a sitting position then move back up, as if you were sitting down on an invisible chair and then standing up again.

THE BASIC HIIT SESSION

Perform each exercise for the required number of repetitions or length of time, then take a 30-second break before starting the next exercise. Repeat this whole process 3–5 times, depending on how fit you are.

Press-up: 10–15 times

If a full press-up is too much, drop your knees to the ground and push up the top half of your body.

Air squats: 15–20 times

As described in the warm up section, perform the sitting to standing motion.

Plank: 45–60 seconds

Get into a prone position, supporting your weight on your toes and forearms. If you need to rest, drop your knees and remember to breathe!

Lunges: 10 on each leg

Stand tall and take a good step forward, then slowly drop your back knee to touch the floor. Keep your body's upright posture throughout. Repeat on the other leg.

High knees: 60 seconds

Sprint on the spot lifting your knees as high as possible.

For some great HIIT ideas, check out Joe Wicks, The Body Coach.

MORNING EXERCISE ROUTINE

Can you spare 15–30 minutes before work to exercise? Or could you get up a little earlier? Your alcohol-free adventure sets up the opportunity to build a solid exercise habit into your life, so why not use the extra energy and improved sleep to create a morning exercise habit?

The advantage of a morning routine is that it will not get pushed out by those unexpected events that happen during the day. Also, your willpower reserves are full, so once you have this habit in place there is no stopping you.

Let's get prepared

Top tip: lay out your kit at the end of the bed every night so you don't have to think about getting it ready in the morning.

Plan your routine

What type of exercise will you perform: running, a HIIT session, yoga, Tai Chi? Make sure it's something you enjoy and will stick with. When you wake up and your self-talk wants to talk you out of it, summon up your willpower and push this to one side.

Reward

The extra energy and vitality produced by your exercise session will have you buzzing all morning. If you do this every day for a week you will start to crave these good feelings and a healthy exercise habit will form without effort.

DAY 11

'IF YOU HAVE HIGH HEART-RATE VARIABILITY, YOU HAVE MORE WILLPOWER AVAILABLE FOR WHENEVER TEMPTATION STRIKES'

KELLY MCGONIGAL [32]

WILLPOWER BOOSTER

A major part of our challenge was gaining the confidence to go against the crowd. As Mark Twain once remarked, 'Whenever you find yourself on the side of the majority, it is time to pause and reflect.' This statement is so true! The vast majority of people we knew believed alcohol was required to have fun, to be successful and to generally enjoy life. Yet we could see the problems that alcohol was bringing to our own lives and those around us. We found ourselves wondering, what if the majority have got it wrong?

Social scientist Solomon Asch performed an incredible experiment during the 1950s, which was designed to test our tendency to follow the crowd, regardless of whether the consensus was wrong. In this test, a group of students was asked to identify which of two lines was the longest. Their answer was predictable: one of the lines was clearly longer than the other. The twist? The majority of participants were actors, prepped beforehand to choose a line that was clearly not the longest.

WOULD THE UNAWARE FOLLOW SUIT?

Amazingly, most of those who weren't prepped would be willing to abandon their own perception in favour of following the group. Social pressure had forced these students to make a decision that went against their better judgement.

Why was this happening? Well, staying part of a group makes sense from an evolutionary standpoint. For early humans, safety came in numbers and life was easier as part of a tribe. In modern life, though, these instincts can be misguided. Being social and having a strong network is vital if you want to flourish, but blindly following suit in situations that are clearly harmful is not beneficial. It takes real courage to take a stand. It is a far braver person who says no to a beer with their mates than one who goes along with the crowd. Fortunately, it only takes one brave person to make a stand to change everything.

Later in his experiment, Asch instructed some of the students to express doubt about the majority's decision. They were prepped to challenge the false answer of the group and to then provide the correct one. This challenge, or polite doubt, gave the 'herd followers' the opportunity they needed to voice their own concerns. In this way, a new consensus was reached and the correct answer agreed upon.

POLITE DOUBT

Non-drinking outliers were our saviours. As we started to question the majority, we began to notice those people who were having wonderfully happy, successful lives without booze. These role models had always been there, but previously they had gone unnoticed by us. Suddenly we found friends, family and sporting heroes who loved life alcohol-free, which gave us the confidence to challenge the majority and make a stand for what we believed in.

This understanding also tells us something powerful about our own actions – that we all have the potential to inspire others to make empowering change. Perhaps by taking this challenge you will inspire a sibling, cousin or friend to change their habits. How cool would that be?

For us, telling people that we were on this alcohol-free challenge was our polite doubt. It offered us a stigma-free opportunity to step away from the herd. Are we geniuses for spotting this? Absolutely not, but it won't be long before millions of others do, and there will be a major shift in thinking that makes it even more cool to be alcohol-free.

Although it might feel daunting to go against the grain right now, it won't be long before the crowd that you are leaving behind will be desperate to get back 'in' with you.

MY HEART IS AFLUTTER

Who would have thought that our heart-rate variability could predict the amount of self-control we have? Heart-rate variability is the interval between one heartbeat and the next. Our heart rate varies all the time throughout the day. When we eat, breathe or run our heart rate moves up and down, and the variability between each heartbeat also moves up and down.

Research suggests that those who have higher variability between heartbeats have more control over their heart rate. For example, this allows them to slow their heart rate more quickly during a stressful event or when faced with temptation. This can lead to reduced stress, increased willpower or control and greater levels of resilience.

When we're under stress our sympathetic nervous system kicks in and puts us into fight or flight mode. In doing so our heart rate jumps and the variability between each heartbeat goes down. In this example, when under stress, the body wants our heart rate to be high to bring on feelings of anxiety and anger in case it is required to fight or flee. It also wants to reduce variability to keep our heart stuck at this higher rate. This is why some people can't calm down once they are in a stressful state. It's in these states that we are more open to temptation. Whereas if someone's heart-rate variability goes up when faced with temptation, they have the control to calm down much more quickly.

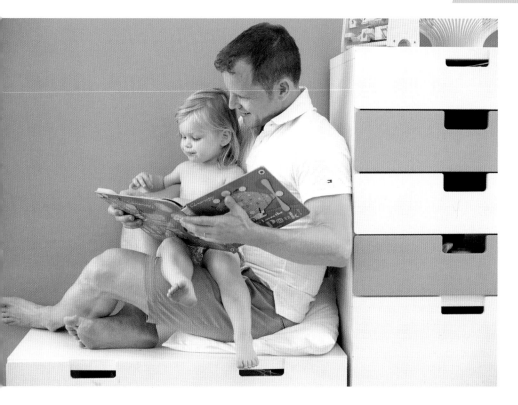

Research shows that people who face their willpower challenges with high heart-rate variability are better at ignoring distraction and delaying gratification[33]. They are also quicker to bounce back after failure and less likely to give up on a willpower challenge. Scientists have been so impressed with these findings that they refer to heart-rate variability as the body's 'reserve' of willpower.

If you imagine that willpower is like a car, those with high heart-rate variability have several gears to move their willpower up and down. Having low variability is like being stuck in one higher gear and not being able to slow down. The more flexible your heart rate, the better you are at adjusting your behaviour to withstand any temptations that might be thrown in your path. The great news is that your heart-rate variability can be improved. Almost every exercise you perform within this challenge will help improve your heart-rate variability. Better sleep, exercise and improved diet will all help to enhance this variability. Mindfulness, which you will practise later in this challenge, is another great way to increase your heart-rate gears.

We love these findings! It's thrilling to discover that by taking this challenge you are actually changing your physiology. As your heart-rate variability increases, so will your willpower to resist temptation – you are gaining a physiological advantage.

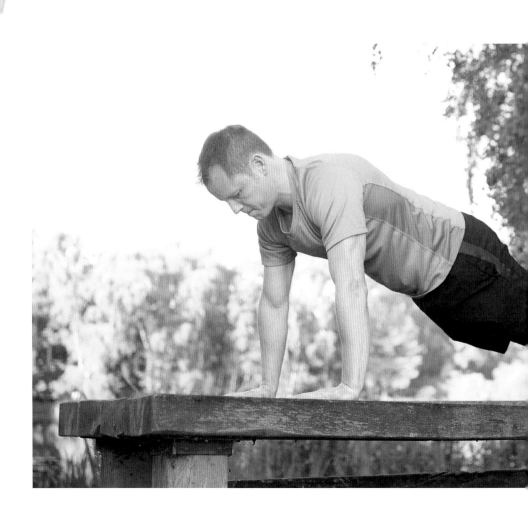

EXERCISE WILLPOWER
BOOSTER

The following exercise will boost both willpower and heart-rate variability. People who practise this breathing technique on a regular basis have reduced stress, cravings and depression. The end result is a sense of relaxed calm that will help you make the right choice in the face of temptation.

The aim of this exercise is to reduce your breathing to four breaths per minute. This is much slower than normal and has an extremely calming effect on the body.

Start by timing your normal breathing, counting how many breaths you take over a one-minute period. Make sure you are sitting comfortably with no distractions.

Then start slowing things down. Most people find that it is easier to slow down on the exhale. Imagine blowing out through a tiny straw, making sure to exhale all the air from your lungs.

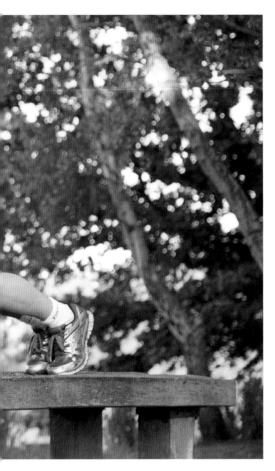

Play around with this exercise, perhaps at different times of day, and see how close to four breaths per minute you can get.

You can download phone apps that will help you with your pacing (see Resources, page 218).

Regular daily practice of this relaxing technique will give you those extra gears to avoid temptation. You can also use this skill before a stressful situation or social occasion that might require a willpower boost.

ALL OR NOTHING

You might be reading this with a belief that this is your last shot at the alcohol-free title. We have seen many members who use this personal threat to motivate them to complete the challenge. Perhaps you have tried many times before and not managed to stay alcohol-free. While we understand this thought process, slip-ups, failure, wagon departures – whatever you want to call them – are an essential learning tool in life. If everyone gave up each time they failed they would achieve nothing.

The story of Shizuka Arakawa, the great ice-skating champion, says it all. While training, she estimated that she fell on her butt more than 20,000 times. That's not one slip-up, that's 20,000, and she kept coming back and learning until she mastered her craft, winning gold at the Winter Olympics in Turin in 2006. Likewise, as quoted on page 72, the basketball legend Michael Jordan told us with pride that he missed 9,000 shots, lost 300 games and on 26 occasions missed the game-winning shot, but he kept learning and coming back for more.

So if you have tripped up a few times, don't allow yourself the easy 'this is my last shot' way out. Why is this your last shot? This is just the start of a learning process on how to be alcohol-free for 28 days (or more) and love it. If you slip up 100 times, who cares? Keep learning and keep coming back stronger until you master the alcohol-free craft.

DAY 12

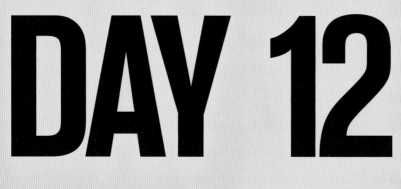

*'DON'T BE
DISHEARTENED
IF YOU HAVE
SETBACKS;
INSTEAD LEARN
FROM THEM AND
ALWAYS CELEBRATE
ANY SUCCESSES.
REMEMBER:
YOU ALWAYS
HAVE A CHOICE'*
PROFESSOR STEVE PETERS [34]

MANAGE YOUR INNER CHIMP FOR LASTING HABIT-CHANGE

The key to a healthy life is habit: eating, exercise and, most importantly, emotional fitness. Habits create a life that enables you to thrive; when the right habits are in place you will not agonise over what food to eat or when to go for a run or how to improve your emotional fitness. You will just do it.

Research has shown that the oldest part of the brain, the basal ganglia, is predominantly responsible for storing habits[35]. This part of the brain existed way back when we were much closer to our primate cousins. This was a time when we acted on instinct, before our rational brain had developed.

Then a few hundred thousand years ago we received a major upgrade. This was not a minor upgrade like moving from an iPhone 5 to a 6; no, this was major overhaul. This upgrade created our new brain, the prefrontal cortex, and developed, amongst other things, willpower.

This new brain made us distinctly human, for suddenly we had the capability to rationalise and use willpower to redirect our primitive instinctual self. When our instinctual self sees cake, it wants to eat it, but thanks to our new brain we have the power to manage this desire.

The key phrase here is 'manage your instinctual self'. Our primitive brain is much more powerful than our newly developed prefrontal cortex. This makes perfect evolutionary sense because the instinctual self is designed to keep us alive long enough to proliferate our genes. To achieve this it will fly in the face of reason to get what it wants.

Professor Steve Peters, the brilliant psychologist behind the British Olympic and Team Sky cycling teams, refers to this older part of the brain as our inner chimp, and the newer more rational part as our inner human. To expand on our previous comments about this on page 31, in his book *The Chimp Paradox* Peters uses this analogy to describe the interaction between these two parts of the brain. The inner chimp or primitive part of our brain, just like a real-world chimp, is much stronger than the newer rational 'human' part. So to achieve effective habit-change we need to learn how to manage our inner chimp effectively rather than fight it, because it will always win in a straight contest.

Problems occur because the old brain stores our habits, hence bad habits are difficult to overcome. On the flip side, if we train our inner chimp with the right habits, it will fight to protect them. For this reason many of the techniques you will try during this challenge are designed to create healthy habits that your inner chimp will happily protect.

QUIT ALCOHOL THE GRATEFUL WAY

Now you might be wondering what on earth gratitude has to do with quitting alcohol? The answer is simple: the act of feeling grateful packs a massive well-being punch. The science behind this claim suggests it's good for your mental and physical health, it helps reduce stress, aids sleep and makes you feel happier[36].

Our mission during this challenge is not just to help you take a break from alcohol, but for you to love life during the time that you are alcohol-free.

 NEGATIVITY BIAS

This exercise is super effective because it begins to reverse our inbuilt negativity bias, which credits more weight to a negative emotion than a positive one. This product of evolution was essential when danger lurked around every corner and worked perfectly when we roamed the savannahs, but is totally outdated in these days of wandering through the supermarket aisles. Our worlds have changed so much since our hunter-gatherer days that for most of us lucky ones there is no longer any real danger to face.

However, our inbuilt negativity bias often misfires, leaving us looking for dangers that no longer exist. Consider this gratitude exercise as an upgrade to your operating system. Over time you will start to notice those things you're grateful for as they happen. This will brighten your day and will counteract the natural pull to the negative, so leaving you feeling more optimistic and happy.

Try this:
Write down three things you're grateful for. It's that simple. It doesn't matter how you make these notes, just so long as you can refer back to them for a well-being boost whenever you need it.

Your reasons for feeling grateful don't need to be huge, they can just be simple things in your life that you feel grateful for.

For example, I am grateful for:

My partner, who made me a lovely meal.
My daughter, who is working hard at school to achieve her goals.
My friend, because his funny story really made me laugh today.

As you conjure these thoughts in your mind, take the time to enjoy the visions. Make them bright and warm and add sound and feelings, if that helps to bring these thoughts to life. Don't rush this process, enjoy recalling these positive feelings. It may seem a little cumbersome at first but please make the effort; it will truly make a difference to your well-being.

For those parents reading this, try this with your children. It is a fantastic way to get them to open up about their day with the bonus of helping them improve their well-being.

HELP! I NEED SOME MOTIVATION

Ok, we understand that not every day is an up day. So if you find yourself underwhelmed or even a little down, here are a few tips to help jolt the motivational system.

1. Remind yourself why you are doing this

Remind yourself of all the reasons why you're here (see page 53).

2. Take a selfie

Take a selfie and compare it with your Day 1 photo. Can you see the difference in your eyes, skin and body?

3. Get social

Check out the OYNB Facebook and forum groups and ask for some help. Or just read some of the inspirational comments.

4. Get moving

Kick-start a change with the motion is emotion exercise (see page 174). Then perform some physical exercise in whatever style you enjoy – walk, run, cycle, do a fitness class, swim or stretch, whatever works for you, but make it happen.

5. The ultimate motivator

There is strong science to indicate that your actions will affect those you love[37]. Remind yourself of all those people close to you who might be positively influenced by this challenge.

6. Do something that makes you happy

This could mean making a nice cup of tea, going shopping or an outing to the theatre. Arrange to do something today that will make you smile inside.

7. Make sure you are eating well

Quality nutrition is key to a healthy mental state. If you forget to eat well today, make some time to consume a really healthy meal as soon as possible.

8. Remind yourself of all the wins

Take a few minutes to remind yourself of all those little victories that have helped you reach this point.

9. Get inspiration from people like you

Finally, check out some of the amazing testimonials throughout the book. These inspirational stories will provide a wonderful motivational boost.

DAY 13

‘NOTHING IN LIFE IS QUITE AS IMPORTANT AS YOU THINK IT IS WHILE YOU'RE THINKING ABOUT IT’

DANIEL KAHNEMAN [38]

MAXIMISE YOUR SOCIAL LIFE

Let's now turn to a Nobel Laureate to discover more about the brain and the peak end rule. How we feel in the moment and how we feel when we reflect on experiences are two different things.

The experiencing self is how you feel at that precise second, when you would be able to answer the question 'Does it hurt now?' This sensation lasts for about three seconds before this moment becomes a memory, at which point your remembering self takes over and would answer the question 'How painful was it on the whole?' So after three seconds, in order to think about an event you have to recall it from memory.

The problem is, the experiencing self has no voice; it's in the moment, then it's gone. Whereas the remembering self holds the power, because once an event has passed, it's this voice that will influence your future actions.

The Nobel Prize-winning psychologist Daniel Kahneman performed a study several years ago during which he profiled the experiences of patients undergoing a painful colonoscopy. (This procedure is no longer painful.) Kahneman discovered that the actual experience and the memory of it produced two completely different results.

During the study patients were continuously asked to rate their pain during the procedure and these results were then mapped to their feelings about the procedure once it was completed.

To Kahneman's surprise, those patients who clearly suffered more pain during the procedure would often report the opposite afterwards, as the pain slowly tapered off towards the end of the procedure. Likewise, those who clearly suffered less pain during the procedure, but felt lots of pain at the very end, reported afterwards that the procedure was much more painful than their pain ratings during the procedure had implied.

This helped Kahneman discover the 'peak end rule'. Put simply, this means that how an experience ends has a big impact on how we remember this experience.

WHY IS THIS IMPORTANT TO OUR CHALLENGE?

We share this knowledge because it shows that our memories can be wrong; they are often distortions of the facts that we create in our heads. So there is an argument that suggests if you keep pushing yourself to be a social alcohol-free hero you might have some less-than-fun experiences at the end of your social events. If this happens too often the peak end rule will kick in and when you reflect on your social events you might believe that they were not much fun, when in truth most of the night was great, it was just at the end that the fun dried up.

This is why we say to cut your nights short when the fun starts to fade. Aim to end all your social events on a high.

YOU HAVE NOTHING TO PROVE

During our first few social occasions we wanted to prove to the world that we still had the same party spirit, even while alcohol-free. So we hit the bars, clubs, late nights and parties, but we quickly discovered that some parts of the night were less fun than others. After a certain time of the evening or drinking session, our friends ended up on a different planet. While it was still a laugh, you can only stand to hear the same story repeated over and over so many times. So rather than force ourselves to be the last man standing, we started to maximise our social occasions up until the point when the fun slowed.

Our advice here would be to plan an exit route, don't say goodbye on your way out unless you have to and don't be afraid to leave when the time feels right. We want you to maximise your social life, to become even more sociable while you're alcohol-free, and using the peak end rule is a great way to paint the best social memories.

With this in mind we entered our social events with a newfound energy. Having released ourselves from the pressure of being a social alcohol-free hero, and knowing that there was a time limit on each event, we set about making the most of these gatherings. Rather than waiting for alcohol to oil the social wheels, we had to make the effort to bring out our A-game, which made our social life much more fun.

Below are a few of our top tips to maximise your alcohol-free social life.

BRING YOUR A-GAME

First and foremost, accept that your social life might change a little and that this challenge is opening up the door to the real you. So psych yourself up before a social event to be on top form. Even if you are not up for it, take a few deep breaths and fake it until you make it. You will be amazed how your state of mind will catch up with your body when you smile and feel alert.

SET UP A MINI CHALLENGE

Try to discover a previously unknown fact about someone within your group – it could be your best mate or a stranger. Take the time to really listen to what they have to say. Give them your full and undivided attention. Hear their words without judgement or trying to give advice; just spark the conversation and let them talk while listening deeply.

Listening is such an underrated social skill and one that alcohol has a tendency to trample all over. We all love to be heard, to be really listened to, because it happens so infrequently. So try listening and asking quality questions to uncover a little more than normal. You might be amazed at what you discover.

If it comes up, don't be afraid to talk about your alcohol-free challenge. Once you overcome the usual knee-jerk social pressure response you will be amazed at how interested people are in discussing not drinking, while drinking. They want to dig deep into your reasons and almost always comment how they would also love to take a break from alcohol. This often leads into some deep conversation that ironically never surfaces when you're both drinking. Enjoy being an expert in these matters. We both

'I had a big birthday dinner out and most of my friends drank that night, but I didn't. The sky didn't come crashing down. I ordered club soda all night long, most people didn't notice, while those who did notice thought it was cool. One of my guy friends, a big drinker himself, ordered club soda to show his solidarity in my birthday drink choice, which was sweet of him. You'll be surprised how well people respond to you not drinking if you give them the chance. I was still raw and wobbly on my birthday so I wasn't ready to talk about my full-stop AF decision. I didn't owe anyone an explanation. We talked about other things. My friends didn't stop being my friends. No one judged, shunned or hassled me then or now for going AF.'

JOLENE

find that some of our best social interactions happen while discussing booze.

MAXIMISE YOUR SOCIAL EVENT

Take five minutes now and use the previous tips to prepare for your next social gathering. Perhaps create a simple plan on paper that lists all those things you can do to maximise this event. The more effort you put in prior to the occasion, the more you will enjoy it. Good luck.

DAY 14

/ 'REMEMBER,
STRESS
EQUALS
FEAR '
TONY ROBBINS [39]

DE-STRESS
WITHOUT ALCOHOL

Alcohol is a well-known depressant[40] and the next day, when you feel groggy or not yourself, anxiety often rears its head. So why on earth do we think that alcohol helps us de-stress? Alcohol also destroys the quality of our sleep, generating more tiredness, which leads to even more stress. We found ourselves caught in the ridiculous cycle of drinking to relieve stress and help us relax, which on waking caused more stress and – guess what? – you feel like you need a drink to help you de-stress and relax.

It was not until we took the time to learn about stress and how to relieve it effectively that we unearthed the truth: alcohol does not relieve stress, it adds to it!

Let's get real here; we can't deny that alcohol, at times, did appear to help our troubles vanish and make us feel more relaxed. But as always there is a price to pay; nothing's for free when it comes to alcohol. This short-term fix did not make our troubles go away, it just drowned them out for a while. On waking, sober and hungover, our problems were 10 times worse.

So we started to explore the alcohol-relaxation connection. When we analysed what was really happening, we discovered the beer after work was just a symbol to say the day was over. It was the couch and being with our loved ones that helped us relax. Alcohol was up to its usual tricks and had convinced us that it was causing these feelings, which in turn created a habit based on false assumptions.

A really clever way to test this theory is to swap your usual alcoholic tipple with a decent alcohol-free version. You will feel relaxed and the beer will still signal the end of the day, but you skip the alcohol.

Prepared with this knowledge we set out to discover activities that really helped us chill. Very soon we had an armoury of different techniques that we could turn to in times of stress without reaching for a beer. Below are just a few:

— **Yoga**
— **Mindfulness**
— **Exercise**
— **Socialising**
— **Cooking**
— **Flow activities such as painting, sport and reading all help you de-stress.**

There are two main differences between these proven activities[41], which will help you to reduce your stress, and drinking. They all require a little more effort than cracking open a beer or bottle of wine. We totally understand this, but this effort is repaid in full because the second and major difference is that they actually reduce your stress long term, not add to it.

DEALING WITH LIFE'S UPS AND DOWNS WITHOUT ALCOHOL IS A POWERFUL THING

When stress was no longer an excuse to drink, we then had to face life head on without the knee-jerk beer. Suddenly our crutch was gone, so surely we would be overwhelmed by a sea of stress that would sweep us away? But rather than our worlds crumbling, the opposite happened – we grew stronger.

It's hard to explain, but there's something really powerful – and empowering – about dealing with all life has to throw at you with a clear head. When we found ourselves in major life situations that historically had had us reaching for a drink – as all around us were losing their composure, usually with alcohol – we were clear-headed and full of focus. Each of these moments enabled us to learn ways to deal with stress – alcohol-free. We grew mentally stronger by the day and rather than stress taking over, it started to fade. We discovered that by removing the alcohol and the hangovers, our stress was reduced. This created – you guessed it – an upward spiral of thriving.

With stress reduced we were in better mental shape to try more stress-busting techniques such as mindfulness and exercise. Each of these improvements, or marginal gains, was leading to more and more small wins – which in turn were making a big impact on our lives and well-being.

So once again, through our own first-hand experience, we smashed the 'alcohol helps me de-stress' myth to pieces.

THE POWER OF SELF-DISCIPLINE

There is a tendency to overlook willpower as a skill you can learn. We are obsessed with the end result: 'I will eat healthily because I want to lose weight or feel better.' While these are great aims, the most praiseworthy part of this regime is missed: self-discipline. Keeping fit, taking a break from alcohol and generally living a healthy life requires a great deal of discipline. So look at things differently and praise yourself for developing the skill of self-discipline rather than waiting for the end result.

LEARNING FROM THE MASTERS

The ancient philosophers were interested in eating healthily and staying fit primarily as a vehicle to practise self-discipline. They put this virtue above any desired outcome of a longer healthier life. They believed there are no guarantees when it comes to health, but the self-discipline required to keep these habits was worthy of praise and kept them on the path to the good life.

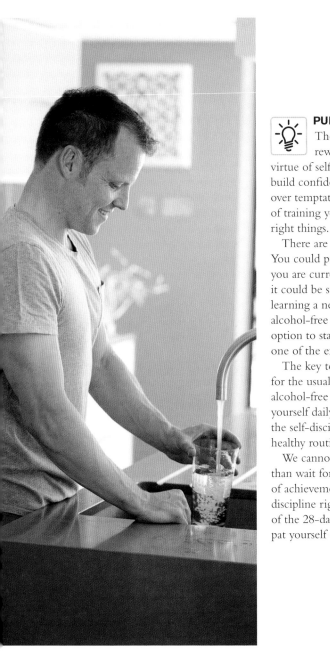

PUMP UP YOUR WILLPOWER

The idea behind this exercise is to reward yourself for displaying the virtue of self-discipline. By doing so you build confidence that you have strength over temptation. This has the added bonus of training your inner chimp to want the right things.

There are two options for this exercise. You could pick an area of your life where you are currently showing self-discipline – it could be sticking to a budget, studying, learning a new language or even this alcohol-free challenge. Or you have the option to start a new routine, perhaps using one of the examples on page 123.

The key to this exercise is not to strive for the usual outcomes, such as staying alcohol-free for a month. Instead, praise yourself daily for staying focused and having the self-discipline to stick with this new healthy routine.

We cannot predict the future, so rather than wait for the end result to feel a sense of achievement, celebrate your show of self-discipline right now. So every day for the rest of the 28-day programme, take 30 seconds to pat yourself on the back for a job well done.

WEEK 2 – REFLECTION

WHAT HAVE YOU OVERCOME?

You have now reached the end of Week 2. So rather than looking ahead, let's celebrate how far you've come by listing a few obstacles you have conquered along the way.

What did you learn? How did you overcome these trials? How have they made you stronger?

These ideas don't have to be massive – it could be resisting wine o'clock or telling your best mate that you are on this challenge. Take five minutes to note down all these ideas. Great effort – you are doing brilliantly.

FILL OUT THE QUICK PROGRESS TRACKER BELOW

Perhaps have a cheeky peek at the results from your pre challenge and Week 1 scores to see if you are making some progress.

Give yourself a rating out of 10 for each of the categories, with 1 being a poor rating and 10 being amazing.

Better yet, record your responses so that you can track your changes over time at **members.oneyearnobeer.com/Test/Week2.**

QUICK PROGRESS TRACKER	
HAPPINESS	/10
MOTIVATION	/10
PRODUCTIVITY	/10
SLEEP	/10
ENERGY	/10
TIME	/10
EXERCISE	/10
OVERALL SCORE	/70

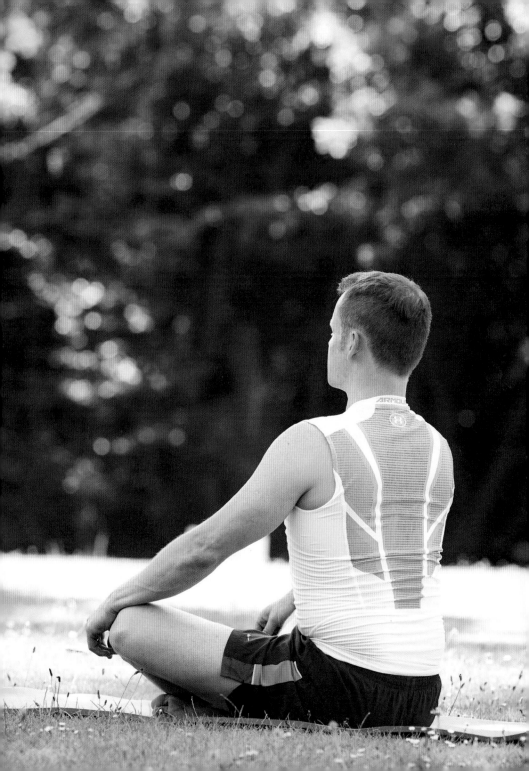

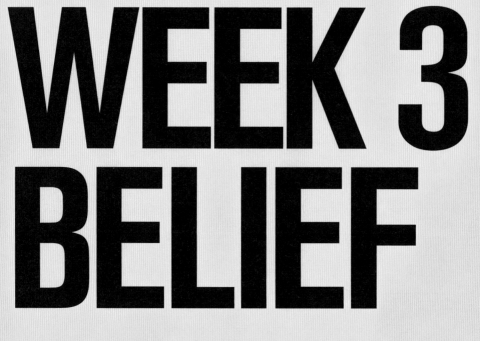

Congratulations, you now have two weeks in the alcohol-free bag and hopefully you're really starting to feel tip-top. As that old-school energy returns, along with the brightness in your eyes, perhaps your relationships are starting to blossom? Loved ones might have noticed the new, improved vibrant you. Perhaps your productivity at work and at home is starting to reach new levels? This is a great week and one that might take you into uncharted alcohol-free territory – and that's when the fun really begins.

As you move into Week 3 you are now starting to build a belief that you can do this, that you can complete this challenge and in doing so make a real difference to your world.

Belief completes the fifth element of habit-change, along with the trigger, routine, reward and craving. Its power is often missed and in our opinion it is the secret ingredient that's required to hack any habit.

So this week is all about creating a belief that what you do matters, while at the same time changing any limiting beliefs you have.

Another key component of habit-change is to be aware of what needs changing. So moving our subconscious routines into our conscious minds is fundamental to positive change. During this week we will also take a look at an amazing awareness tool called mindfulness. This technique will help you surf the urge to overcome cravings and create space between stimulus and response.

DAY 15

‹WHETHER YOU
THINK YOU CAN,
OR YOU THINK
YOU CAN'T –
YOU'RE RIGHT›
HENRY FORD [42]

BELIEVE IN YOURSELF

Beliefs can change in an instant, but without awareness of what needs to be changed, nothing can happen. Hopefully you are starting to see a pattern emerging. By cultivating awareness you can decide which beliefs and habits you want to keep and in doing so you can change your world.

Your beliefs have the power to create a wonderful existence but equally to create one of misery and suffering.

A belief is a statement or a feeling that you 'believe' to be true. You build these beliefs over time – often through personal experience – and they help shape the way you interact with the world.

Many of our deep-seated beliefs come not from our direct experience, but as hand-me-downs from parents, religions or other influential people in our lives. These are the types of beliefs we don't question, we just believe it is right because it is. Often there is truth in these ideals, but not always; therefore it's important to question for yourself why you feel the way you do. If something is upsetting you, ask why. Why do I feel this way? Often you will find it's due to a belief that was given to you by someone else.

One of the great side-effects of undertaking an alcohol-free challenge is to highlight that long-held beliefs such as 'You need alcohol to have fun' are limiting your world and holding you back. Just because you have held a belief for a long time does not mean it cannot be challenged and changed. A key message here is that you can

decide what to believe and by doing so you can influence the way you feel.

FIND AND CHANGE A BELIEF

Take 10 minutes to think about your personal beliefs. Note down as many as you can. Then take a step back and decide if these beliefs are helpful or not.

Group them into positive and negative beliefs. Try to remember where these beliefs came from. Are they hand-me-downs from a parent or friend? Or are they experiences you had in the past?

Examples of positive beliefs:

'My family will support me no matter what.'
'I have the courage to bounce back.'
'I can learn to change my habits.'

Examples of negative beliefs:

'Everyone knows I have zero willpower.'
'I will never stick to a diet.'
'I can't compete with these guys.'

Enjoy this process as you start to become aware of what's in your mind. Once you bring these thoughts into your consciousness, you can decide if you want to keep these beliefs or change them. This is how you weed the garden of your mind.

Often it is our subtle beliefs that cause the most harm. Your aim is to highlight and support your positive beliefs while undermining and breaking down any negative ones.

CHANGE A BELIEF

If you find a belief that is holding you back, the first thing to do is take away its power. For example, if you hold a belief that says 'I cannot socialise without alcohol', write this statement out on a piece of paper and challenge it until the power melts.

Ask yourself these sort of questions:

- **Is it helpful to believe in this statement? Is it making your world better?**

- **Has there ever been a time that you have socialised without alcohol?**

- **Did you socialise without alcohol when you were younger?**

- **Do you have social interactions that don't involve alcohol?**

Imagine you are a top-shot lawyer and it is your job to destroy this unfounded belief. Keep performing this process with each and every belief that is holding you back.

BUILD A BELIEF

The way to build a belief is through daily small actions. For example, every day that you remain alcohol-free builds a firm belief that you can thrive without alcohol. This is our aim to help you smash all those limiting beliefs around alcohol and then build a new empowering belief that you no longer need it. You can use this same understanding to build other healthy beliefs, such as, you are a person who exercises every day.

To make this happen you need to support this belief on a daily basis using small actions. So in this example you would aim to exercise every day. But here's the thing; this does not have to mean a massive gym session or even a HIIT workout. You could include jogging on the spot for five minutes or using the stairs at work instead of the lift. The key is to complete some form of exercise every day even if it is only for a few minutes. This will train you to believe that you are the sort of person who exercises every day. Once the belief grows you can create a more adventurous exercise plan, safe in the knowledge that you will subconsciously want to make every session to maintain this new belief.

IF YOU MISS A DAY DON'T WORRY, JUST DO IT THE NEXT DAY

Science has also shown that missing the odd day does not materially affect habit formation[43]. Imagine that each positive action is casting a vote for this new belief

RUARI'S STORY

Have you ever had one of those moments when you come across a group of people who share a similar passion for something that you had no idea existed? This happened to me recently after I decided to head to the woods for an early morning walk. On turning a corner I was confronted with a sea of bright colours – people young and old, babies in prams and dogs on leads. Struggling to get my head around this eclectic mix, which appeared like some sort of organised race, I

approached one of the marshals to find out more. The young man's exuberant smile and genuine enthusiasm shone through as he explained that this was a Parkrun – a free, timed 5k event – held every Saturday at 9 a.m. all over the world in local parks to get people moving. You can walk, sprint, bring the dog or run with a pram. No one comes last; it's the taking part that counts. He went on to explain that he volunteers because he loves being a part of a group that is

*coming together once a week, to be outdoors, enjoy nature and do something really positive in their lives.
This brief encounter opened my eyes to a new world of people who, only minutes before, I had no idea even existed. What a beautiful idea! I could be a part of this community, bring my wife and daughters and kick-start our weekends as a family in the most positive of ways.*

and each time you don't exercise is a vote against, but as long as you receive enough votes for your new belief, this will stick.

DISCOVERING A NEW TRIBE

One of the great joys in life is being part of a tribe that supports your aims and dreams. When we first looked at going alcohol-free we could not find such a tribe, so we decided to create our own. This inspirational group motivates us on a daily basis to continue on this alcohol-free adventure.

Make sure you have joined the oneyearnobeer tribe at www.oneyearnobeer. com – we are waiting for you!

Just like the story above, when you first start your alcohol-free adventures you discover a tribe of people that you

probably never noticed before. There is a real opportunity to be part of a new crowd, one that's trying something exciting and really positive. It is within this new tribe that you can flip the social pressure and use it to your advantage. So if you haven't already joined the OYNB group, do so now and become a part of this inspirational tribe.

'Thank you EVERYONE here for all your support – couldn't have even dreamt of it without this group. 60 here I come!'

CLARICE

DAY 16

AWARENESS SHINES A LIGHT ON OUR HABITS

Too many people are running through life on autopilot, driven by habits and a conditioning that they don't question. They just do stuff, because that's what they have always done. Never stopping to consider if the things they are doing are good for them, or if these things are making them unhealthy, both physically and emotionally.

A key part of this challenge is to bring awareness into your life, which will allow you to take an objective view of things as they really are. This switches off the autopilot and allows you to decide, in full conscious control, if your habits are helping or hindering.

From awareness comes the ability to change. You have shown great awareness by starting this challenge, and now we want to build on this. Try this quick exercise.

For the next two minutes, close your eyes and relax. Feel your breathing slowing down as you start to loosen up.

Notice your thoughts as they come and go. Is your head full of noise, ideas and things to do? Or is it pretty chilled? There are no wrong or right answers in this exercise; we are simply looking for awareness of what's going on right now in this moment.

Try listening to your breathing as the air flows in and out of your lungs. Breathe in through your nose and out through your mouth. Stay with this as long as you can.

If your mind starts to chase a story, bring your attention back to the breath. (Head to oneyearnobeer.com/book-resources for an audio version of this exercise.)

This exercise usually throws up one major learning point: keeping your mind focused on something as simple as breathing is pretty tough. The mind wants to wander all the time. But this constant mind travel is often the cause of stress and worry over things that have not happened or have already gone.

How many times has an issue from work followed you home? How many times have you missed a smile or a comment from a loved one because you are dealing with a problem from the past in your head? Or how many times have you worried about an event that never actually occurred later?

When we run on autopilot, mindlessly chasing every story, we miss the beauty of the present moment. The practice you just performed is designed to keep your attention on the present moment so you can appreciate what's going on – right now. You may have recognised that this was a mindfulness meditation practice. We deliberately avoided labelling this exercise to allow you to have the experience without preconceptions. Over the course of the challenge you will learn more about this powerful habit-change tool and how you can create many more first-hand experiences.

HEALTHY WARNING

It is easy to feel that you understand mindfulness and then either dismiss it as not for you or never really experience its potential. Please stick with these exercises until you have fully understood this practice – it might just change your life.

Think of mindfulness as mental training. We know we have to train our bodies to be physically fit, and mindfulness training keeps us emotionally fit. Just like physical exercise, the more you practise mindfulness the fitter you become.

WHAT EXACTLY IS MINDFULNESS?

Mindfulness is the skill of being aware of the present moment in our daily lives. By bringing attention to the here and now without making judgements we can learn to appreciate the beauty of the present moment. This helps us to control our minds, preventing them from rushing into the future and back to the past. Mindfulness is much more than a formal practice, it is an attitude to life that is something worth aiming to cultivate at all times.

WHAT IS MEDITATION?

Meditation is the formal practice of training our minds to be more aware of the present moment and therefore mindful. This can be done in many ways; from the classic sitting pose to walking, running, swimming, washing the dishes – the options are endless. As long as there is a purposeful effort to focus on the present moment without judgement, then you are training your brain to be more mindful.

WHY IS MINDFULNESS SO IMPORTANT TO HABIT-CHANGE?

To change a habit you must first be aware of it. Mindfulness creates a powerful awareness that brings subconscious routines into your conscious mind. From this point you can decide which habits you want to change. Also, awareness of your actions can create a tiny space between stimulus and response. Within this space you can make conscious decisions that fit your goals – for example, to avoid alcohol – rather than be dragged around by subconscious unhealthy habits and cravings. On Day 21 we will show you a mindfulness exercise to overcome cravings called 'surfing the urge' (see page 158).

WHAT ARE THE MAIN BENEFITS OF MINDFULNESS?

The science-backed benefits of mindfulness[45] are almost overwhelming. Mindfulness has been shown to:

— **Reduce cravings**

— **Help increase our habit-changing friend – heart-rate variability**

— **Boost self-confidence and self-acceptance**

— Decrease stress, anxiety, depression

— Enhance well-being; it makes people happier and brings more meaning into people's lives

— Bolster positive emotions such as hope, optimism and gratitude

— Improve your physical body by reducing blood pressure and heart rate, and when combined with traditional medicine, it produces better results.

All these findings are backed by strong scientific data. Far from needing to spend a lifetime in a monastery, studies have shown that within just a few weeks of regular practice many of these benefits will kick in.

IS MY HEAD SUPPOSED TO TOTALLY CLEAR OF THOUGHTS?

No, your conscious mind will always generate thoughts. You are not trying to stop them, you are simply trying to watch them from a distance without creating big stories from these tiny ideas.

DO YOU HAVE TO SIT ON A CLOUD WHEN PERFORMING THE FORMAL PRACTICE?

No, you can sit any way you want as long as you are both relaxed and alert, whatever that means to you.

I DON'T GET MUCH TIME TO SIT, CAN YOU PRACTISE IN ANY OTHER WAYS?

Yes! Once you have the basic skills, the aim is to bring mindfulness into all areas of your life: mindful walking, eating, washing the dishes and waiting for the bus/train. The idea is always the same, to be present in the moment rather than letting your mind wander into the past or future.

I DON'T THINK I AM VERY GOOD AT MINDFULNESS. CAN YOU HELP?

Firstly, you can't have a bad or good meditation; you are simply aiming to be mindful of the present moment. Sometimes your mind will settle easily and other times it will be full of noise and take time to slow down. Don't worry, just sit, observe your thoughts and see what comes up.

I WANT TO KNOW MORE – WHAT SHOULD I DO?

Our aim is to introduce you to the basics of mindfulness during this challenge, but this is a wide and varied topic that we recommend you explore outside the boundaries of this book. See Resources (page 218) for further reading, recommended apps and courses.

You can listen to our free meditations by visiting our main website: www.oneyearnobeer.com/book-resources

DAY 17

'IF YOU BELIEVE YOU CAN CHANGE – IF YOU MAKE IT A HABIT – THE CHANGE BECOMES REAL'

CHARLES DUHIGG [46]

GENERATE GOOD HABITS, THEY WILL PUSH OUT THE BAD

'EVERYONE HAS A PLAN UNTIL THEY GET PUNCHED IN THE FACE.'
MIKE TYSON [47]

Mike Tyson's brilliant quote sums up life perfectly. You can plan, you can prepare and then – just when you think everything is under control – bam! You get (metaphorically) punched in the face. It is in these moments that your character and resilience are tested. Life is so unpredictable that you never know when this might happen.

Be prepared for the stray left hook. It could be an old friend arriving back in town who wants to meet for a drink, or an unexpected invitation to the ball. During your challenge, things will happen out of the blue that will test you. Be ready. Remember, you knew this would happen. Remind yourself of your long-term goals and how great you feel right now, and refocus on your major aim of completing this challenge alcohol-free.

Each time you overcome one of these random obstacles you will grow stronger, building resilience and resources that will help you weather life's blows.

See the friend and accept the invite, but be strong and make it clear you will do it – without the beer.

WHAT GOES DOWN MUST COME UP

Is there such a thing as a happiness set point or a well-being baseline? Or a level of well-being that dictates how you feel most of the time? The evidence suggests there is and, what's more exciting, it also suggests that through our own efforts we can move this baseline higher [48].

Adaptation is an interesting concept that lends itself to a happiness baseline theory. To experience moments of joy and ecstasy, our level of happiness needs to move up. What goes up must come down, thus allowing us to experience these highs again at a later date. This is why there is no happiness Nirvana where we can feel 100 per cent happy all the time. This would leave us with nowhere to go and life would become dull. For most people, our predisposed level of happiness is mildly happy – let's say six out of 10 – and it's from here that we experience the joys of life.

The wonderful part about adaptation is that it works both ways. When we experience upset and trauma the same adaptation drags us from feeling low back to our baseline of mildly happy. This is our psychological immune system kicking in. We have to get over these traumas in order to keep going.

Some exciting research shows that we can move this well-being baseline higher. So there is an opportunity to start your days feeling even better, for example, moving from a six to perhaps an eight out of 10.

The beauty of this challenge is that many of the skills you are learning will raise your happiness and well-being baseline. Breaking pessimistic thoughts, increasing optimism, building strong social bonds, taking a break from alcohol, exercising more often and many other actions all help to do this. As we have consistently discovered, taking a break from alcohol is often the keystone habit that unlocks many of the well-being benefits above. This in turn helps move your baseline a little higher – how cool is that? So throw yourself into the exercises and keep building on your healthy lifestyle – you might become a little happier in the process.

 GENERATE GOOD HABITS – THEY WILL SOLVE THE BAD

Now that you understand how the habit loop works, let's use this knowledge to create some new healthy habits. The idea is simple: by creating more good habits you will push out the bad. This is why so many members experience total life transformations as each healthy habit builds on the next to create a positive upward spiral.

Take exercise. You may have decided that going to a spin class once a week is good for you, and you're right, it is. So don't question the merits of this activity; it will help you to get fit, lose weight, you will feel good about yourself and your well-being will be boosted.

Science has shown us that habits require a trigger, routine and reward. To build good habits, make sure all three pieces of the habit puzzle are present.

Step one:
Create your cue: a regular day and time
Your brain likes routine, so to help build a solid habit try to arrange a regular time and place for this to take place. For example, 7:30 a.m. every Monday is your trigger. There is no thinking about it, or booking at the last minute. You can plan your diary knowing that this time is spoken for. This is a key concept – once you agree that a habit is good for you, the trick is to hammer this routine into your subconscious. Plan ahead, if you have to, and book the class, knowing that every week at this time you will be exercising. This helps take away the brainwork; you do not need to think about it or question its merits, you know it's good for you. All you have to do is turn up, pump the pedals, love the burn and reap the rewards.

Don't think – just do.

Step two:
Create the routine

In this example we used a spin class but it could be any form of exercise that you enjoy. Run, swim, walk, dance … whatever activity sparks joy.

Step three:
Add in a reward

At the end of your exercise routine you will be full of endorphins and will feel great for having made the effort. If a tangible reward is required, refer back to Day 2 to make sure the reward is in keeping with your goals. For example, if you like to be rewarded with social interaction, book a group class or exercise with friends. As you learn about your world you will become more efficient and will design it to meet your needs and in doing so create a vibrant lifestyle.

Step four:
Crave your reward

Craving closes the habit loop. The sense of achievement you get from exercise alone is addictive and you will crave the so-called 'runner's high'. You will look better, feel better, have more energy and crave these wonderful feelings. Also, if you decided to select a specific reward this will ignite craving, which will feed the habit and close the loop.

THEY BREED LIKE HABITS

Let's make baby habits. Use the headings below to sketch out a healthy habit that you would like to develop; one that will guide you towards your goals. Make sure you fill out all parts of the habit loop. This will help you create a permanent empowering baby habit.

Cue

Wake up, walk into kitchen, put porridge in microwave.

Routine

Grab yoga mat, put on timer for 10 minutes. Slow meditational yoga.

Reward

Back and joints feel alive and less stiff. Feeling calm yet awake.

Craving

Feeling supple, wanting to stretch out the body. Back less sore and stiff.

Use this rough format to design more empowering habits. Keep them simple - your brain likes it that way.

BELIEVE IN YOUR NEW HABITS

The final piece of the puzzle is embracing the belief that you have the power to change. Each time you hack a habit you will be more confident that what you do matters. This is such an important part of well-being.

DAY 18

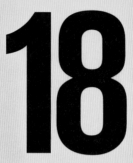

'IT IS A ROUGH
ROAD THAT
LEADS TO THE
HEIGHTS OF
GREATNESS'
SENECA [49]

THE CROSSROADS OF LASTING CHANGE

Entertaining clients (with plenty of alcohol on hand) oils the wheels of business – at least, that's what we've been led to believe. From construction workers to dentists, being social and entertaining clients with alcohol often equates to climbing the corporate ladder. We cannot dress this up and pretend it's not so.

A major worry for us was that if we stopped drinking while entertaining clients we would lose our edge, our business and ultimately our income. This is a scary thought and one that can keep people in a negative cycle.

Once alcohol-free, however, we discovered that our productivity went through the roof, and our clients were happier with a service that did not ebb and flow around hangovers.

Pretty soon we smashed the myth that alcohol was required when meeting clients and socialising. We both experienced a double win: business was up and expenses were down. Also another interesting thing happened – we were forced to rework the usual drinks nights. We had to adapt and create different ways to socialise. Clients loved the extra effort and experiences we were offering. We formed deeper bonds and business skyrocketed in ways we never thought possible.

There will be those of you reading this who are thinking, 'Well, in my industry you NEED to drink.' But we can assure you that's what we once thought too and through our own experiences we have smashed that limiting belief.

LET'S BREAK THE BRAVADO

Another alcohol myth is the assumption that everyone wants to drink. We are convinced that if you could read people's minds at many 'social' functions, the majority would prefer not to drink but are all caught in the same trap: 'If they are drinking, I must follow suit. I can't be seen to be the only one not drinking.'

Not long after we started our challenge, we began to notice this beer pressure all around us. We saw it at work functions, nights out with the lads and Sunday afternoon gatherings. It was everywhere. Yet when we started to resist and do something different by not drinking, we noticed a common pattern: more and more people were choosing to join us. It was as though we had given them the excuse they were looking for – they just needed someone else to have the courage to ditch the booze.

Imagine the scenario: three people are meeting for dinner and none of them wants to drink. One has an exercise class booked in the morning, the other left the car at the train station, and the third person is totally over the hangovers.

As they enter the restaurant they're apprehensive about the direction the evening will take. The dream is that it will be alcohol-free. Yet the social pressure weighs heavy. Like a nuclear strike they wait. Fingers poised on the red button. No one wants this; they know the damage it will do, but they must react to protect their status.

Waiter

'What would you like to drink?'

Drinker #1 thinks

They are going to think I am such a wuss if I order water, but I really want to make the early exercise class. Why, oh why, do I have to be the first to order? I bet they're dying for a drink. Oh sod it − *'I'll have a beer, please.'*

Drinker #2

Nightmare, exactly what I didn't want! If he is having one, then I can't wimp out.
'I'll have one as well.'

Drinker #3

I can't be the only one on the water!
'Perfect, that suits me, I'll have a beer.'

Why are we so weak? We all like to think we are tough, but we crumble in this way all the time.

Let's play this scenario again:

Waiter

What would you like to drink?

Drinker #1

There is no way I am missing my class. I don't care what the others think, it takes a real hero to say no!
'I'm fine with water, please.'

Drinker #2

Phew, disaster avoided!
'I have one as well.'

Drinker #3

What a result!
'Perfect, that suits me, I'll have water.'

Of course, this is not always the case, but on so many occasions it is. So let's break this bravado; it's not big and it's not clever. It takes a real man or woman to say no. When you next find yourself in a similar situation, remember this exercise. Stay strong and stick to your guns. Order the non-alcoholic option, because for all their bravado, those around you are probably looking for an excuse to do exactly the same!

THE CROSSROADS

This exercise will provide extra motivation towards a specific goal. Find a goal or aim where you feel you need some extra help. Whether it's to lose a certain amount of weight, stop smoking, run a marathon or complete this alcohol-free challenge, the same principles apply.

In this example we will focus on completing your alcohol-free challenge.

Begin by relaxing your body and mind, taking five long deep breaths in through your nose, then slowly breathing out through your mouth. Now that you're feeling relaxed, let's begin.

Take five minutes to perform this exercise:

Close your eyes and imagine yourself at the crossroads of life; you can build an image of a crossroads in your mind. Perhaps you can see two old country lanes with a white signpost pointing in each direction. One leads to the road of no change, while the other points to the road of total control.

We would like you to take the road of no change first.

As you walk down this road, visualise your life six months from now, having not made any positive changes in your world, having not achieved your intended goal to take a break from alcohol. How do you feel, how does your body look? Take some time to create a vivid picture – the more feeling you add the more powerful it will be. Add colour, sound, feeling, make it bigger and really go to town. How does it feel to still be drinking? Are your loved ones pleased? Are you disappointed with yourself? Ask these questions of yourself, build up some emotional discomfort.

Ok that's enough of that, now bring yourself back to the crossroads and shake off the unpleasant feelings you just created. If possible we would advise physically shaking that feeling out of your body, as if you were shaking down before exercise.

Now follow the sign that says you are 28 days alcohol-free. Again, make this a bright colourful picture. How do you feel? How do you look? Who are you with? What are you doing? How has your life changed? Build a compelling vision of yourself. We bet this feels great; don't rush this experience, revel in the new you, enjoy having achieved so much.

When you are ready, come back to the signpost and look at both paths – 'Nothing's changed' or '28 days alcohol-free'. Which one do you want to take?

You can perform this exercise with each of your goals as many times as necessary to gain the emotional leverage required to succeed.

DAY 19

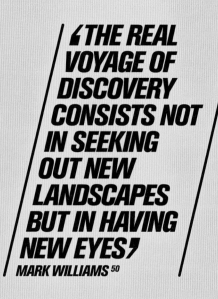

'THE REAL VOYAGE OF DISCOVERY CONSISTS NOT IN SEEKING OUT NEW LANDSCAPES BUT IN HAVING NEW EYES'

MARK WILLIAMS [50]

MINDFULNESS ON THE GO

**Many years ago, as an army approached a Buddhist monastery, the monks were frightened that the soldiers would steal their prized statue of a golden Buddha. So they quickly covered the Buddha in concrete and mud to make it look like an old grey statue.
As the army plundered the village they gazed upon the statue and, thinking it worthless, left it alone. For years the village remained in the hands of these rebels, and as time passed people forgot about the Golden Buddha.**

Then one day a monk who was meditating at the foot of the Buddha noticed a small crack in the statue. On closer inspection he could see something bright inside. Intrigued, he picked at the crack and a piece of concrete fell to the ground revealing a truth that had been hidden for many years - the Buddha was golden.

This wonderful metaphor reminds us of our relationship with alcohol. Over time, society and conventional wisdom make us forget what it feels like to be alcohol-free. We forget how much brighter and more productive our lives were before we started drinking. We forget what it feels like to have our natural energy back, along with a decent night's sleep. We forget that we can enjoy our social lives alcohol-free and reclaim our morning motivation.

Then one day a crack appears and we experience a taste of life alcohol-free. From this moment on we know the truth – that life was golden after all.

MINDFULNESS ON THE GO

You can practise mindfulness anywhere and everywhere – even while multi-tasking. The more we are aware of our actions, the better chance we have to correct and change our habits. The real power of mindfulness is that it brings conscious control into our daily routines.

Today we want to bust a mindfulness myth and show you that in order to practise you do not need to sit on a cloud while chanting 'om'. You can practise mindfulness anywhere and everywhere while you are performing all sorts of daily tasks.

This forms a double win: as you practise you become more aware of your habits, which allows you to pick and choose the ones you want to keep.

Also, by experimenting with various types of practice you will find a style that you enjoy. For some people the thoughts of sitting and watching their breath might hold little appeal. They might prefer to walk, feeling their feet against the ground or listening to the noise of daily life.

There are no wrongs or rights, just as long as you are bringing deliberate focused attention to the here and now, then you are practising mindfulness.

Below are some examples of how you can practise mindfulness meditation on the go:

— Running
Focus on your breathing and/or bodily sensations.

— Walking
Focus on your feet as they touch the earth below. Perhaps listen to the noise of life in the present moment.

— Swimming
Focus on your breathing and/or the sensations of the water as you glide.

— Washing the dishes
Focus on the temperature of the water, the noise of the dishes and clean fragrances.

— Showering
Focus on the water as it collides with your body, notice how this feels.

— Brushing your teeth
Focus on the sensations of the brush as it moves around your mouth. Notice the taste and smell of the toothpaste and how this makes your mouth feel.

You get the idea, you can practise mindfulness meditation anywhere – so there is no excuse not to try! As long as you are staying with the present moment, in the here and now, in a non-judgemental fashion, you are exercising your mind muscles. As your mind muscles strengthen so will your awareness, which will help you make the right choice when faced with temptation, guiding you to challenge victory.

THE NON-JUDGEMENTAL APPROACH

When you practise mindfulness a key concept to grasp is that of a non-judgemental approach. This means that you avoid weighing up every thought as good or bad. When you make judgements about a thought as it enters your head this often leads you into the story of the thought and away from the present moment.

For example, when a thought pops up about a work deadline, there is a tendency to weigh this up as good or bad. If we are behind schedule it's bad, leaving us feeling anxious and worried. The mind then wants to create stories around this. You might imagine getting into trouble with the boss, letting your colleagues down or, worse still, getting fired. Pretty quickly this tiny thought, when evaluated as good or bad, has turned into a major stressful event.

The mindful way is to acknowledge these thoughts as they enter your head, but not to judge them. They are just thoughts – that's it.

ANDY'S STORY

When I first started practising mindfulness and bringing awareness into my life I stumbled upon a couple of startling revelations. For the last six years, on my way to work, I had always entered the train station and turned right, because this was the end nearest my destination exit. I would complain daily that I could never get a seat and would often end up sardined into a tiny space. Then one day something strange happened. I turned off autopilot and realised that I was playing this same routine every day. So feeling brave and in full awareness, I entered the station and turned left. For me this was unchartered territory. In six years I had never turned left and here I was at the wrong end of the train. As the train pulled in my heart raced. I was apprehensive, almost scared as to what would await me. The doors flung open and there before me was a sight I had not seen in six years. An empty seat!

The real power of mindfulness is that it helps us turn off autopilot for long enough to notice what's really happening in our worlds. Once you have this awareness you can start to make changes to your habitual routines. You can tweak and enhance the good ones, while replacing the habits that hold you back.

This does not mean they are the truth, they are just ideas that the brain produces. When you get to grips with this, you will discover that you have the choice to follow these thoughts or not.

A key point is that these thoughts can't predict the future or make things happen, they are just thoughts on a subject.

The greatest gift of mindfulness is that it gives you a choice of how you want to react, which is why it is so important to habit-change. You will gain the ability to see your thoughts or cravings from a distance in a non-judgemental fashion, and from this point make the choice that is right for you and your goals.

During your practice, try imagining your thoughts as boats gently floating down a river, as you sit and watch from the river's edge. You are not trying to climb aboard each boat to take control, you are quietly sitting and admiring the view while passing no judgement about each boat as it gently drifts by.

The next exercise starts to build on these ideas by bringing a mindful approach to your morning routine.

MINDFUL MORNING EXERCISE

For the remainder of this week try to start your day mindfully. Create a reminder on your alarm, if this helps. Rather than letting your mind run on autopilot as you prepare for work, make a conscious effort to stay in the moment. Enjoy the sounds of morning, or the quiet it brings. Feel the water as it runs down your back in the shower, the brush against your teeth. Listen for the sounds of the birds above you or the cars as they pass.

Perhaps try to notice as many things as you can on your walk to work.

This is often when we're in full autopilot mode – racing to the office with a head full of tasks and concerns. Try staying with your breath and notice as much as you can about your journey. Perhaps you pass some flowers or gardens you never noticed before, or you might hear the birds singing. Mix up your routine, sit on a different seat or use a new part of the train or park the car somewhere different. The idea is to shake up your subconscious routines and bring them into the full spotlight of awareness. This is going to help you change your habits around alcohol and give you the control you need to build new healthy routines.

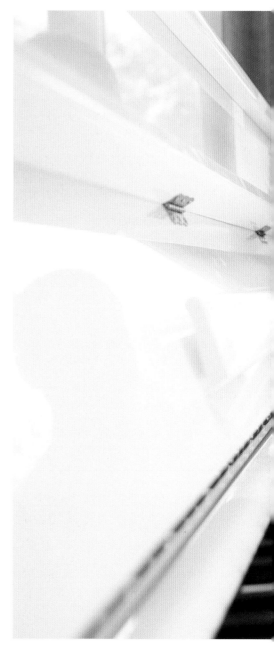

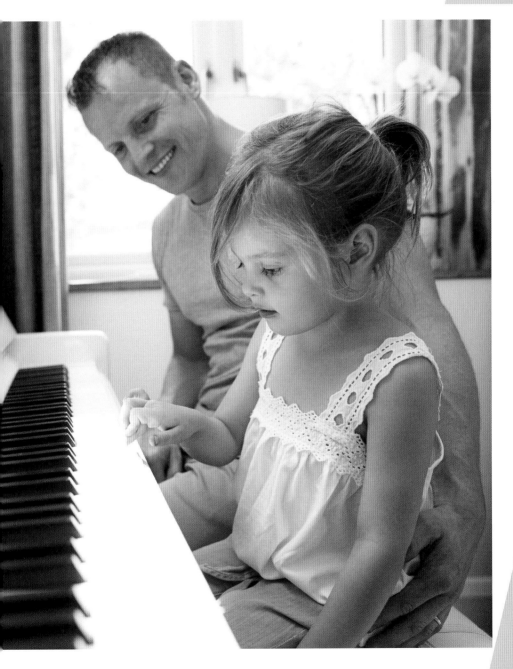

DAY 20

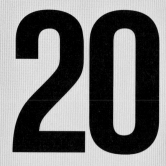

‘MEN ARE
DISTURBED
NOT BY THINGS,
BUT BY THE
VIEW WHICH
THEY TAKE
OF THEM’
EPICTETUS [51]

YOU AND YOU ALONE ARE RESPONSIBLE FOR THIS CHANGE

More than 2,000 years ago the great Greek philosopher Epictetus told us that we have total control to decide how we feel. Just sit with this for a while. You have total and full control to decide how you feel. It's not what's happening in the world around us that matters, only what we decide that counts. This is why some people can thrive in the most dire of circumstances while others suffer when they appear to have it all. Life is a mental game.

The ancient philosophers understood years ago what we still wrestle with today, which is this: the only thing really under our control is our emotions. Beyond our emotions, everything else, to a more or less extent, is out of our full control. So we should not concern ourselves over things we cannot fully influence. Fame and fortune can come and go, our loved ones might end up loving someone else, jobs and security can vanish overnight. When you really reflect on most objects, people and things you realise that they are all, to a degree, out of our control. But the real power comes from controlling your own emotions; it is through this lens that we see the world. If you can control the way you feel, you can control your beliefs, and in doing so control your world. This puts all the power into your hands. This is such an important understanding and one that can totally change the way you view things.

It's an extremely powerful message and in many ways leaves you nowhere to hide.

You cannot blame your feelings on the government, job, partner or luck. There is only one person who can decide how you feel, and that is you. You have full control to decide what you feel about a particular situation, which in turn will control your beliefs towards the same event.

POWER UPS

Another mindfulness myth is that it means dropping out or losing your competitive edge. We have heard people worry that meditating will get in the way of them being productive – when the opposite is true.

As the day progresses, we accumulate more and more stress, which can lead to what science calls 'emotional and cognitive overload'. If you can imagine opening more and more apps on your smartphone over the course of the day – eventually it will start to slow down until it runs out of memory. It is the same with our brains. Over the course of a stressful day we build up more and more emotional and cognitive load, which slows us down. So we end up with less storage to complete those technical tasks.

This is why mindfulness can enhance our productivity and reduce stress, which will help you stay on the path to challenge glory. Mindfulness can clear all the apps that are running in the background and wipe clean this cognitive load. This allows us to work harder, for longer, at full efficiency throughout the day, because our brains don't get overloaded.

Try the 'power up' exercise below to remain super productive and keep stress at bay.

During your day take just 60 seconds once an hour, if possible, to reconnect with the present moment.

Wherever you are or whatever you are doing, find some space to relax. Feel your body loosen and your cheeks go soft. Let your eyebrows feel nice and smooth and soften your face.

Breathe into your body and with each out breath feel more relaxed. Keep your mind on the present moment. Perhaps focus on your breath or your body as it relaxes.

Keep this going for at least one minute.

A top tip here is to set an alarm on your phone to go off every hour. You can label it 'Power Up' as a gentle reminder to perform this refreshing exercise.

The real power behind this technique is that it reconnects us with the present moment. As our days progress we often get so entangled in the stress of life that we live and breathe this stress and anxiety. This power up breaks the cycle, allowing us to see clearly once more and take a step back from what is it we are doing so that we can, once again, form an objective view. From this vantage point we can make the choices that are in keeping with our goals, while avoiding temptation.

YOU AND YOU ALONE ARE RESPONSIBLE FOR THIS AMAZING CHANGE

If you are feeling a mid-challenge malaise, remind yourself that you and you alone are responsible for this positive change. It takes a lot of courage to go against the social grain and take on a challenge such as this. Take huge pride in the fact that you are being proactive and giving yourself a shot at the well-being title.

There are so many people out there who are waiting for someone or something to force their hand. They secretly wish for some awful event – the break up, the job loss, the illness or the threat – to happen to them, which will take away all responsibility for change.

You are different, you have taken this challenge on for yourself. It is a bold step to accept full responsibility for your own actions. There is only one person who can stop you completing this challenge, and that is you. This very same person is also the only one who can help you succeed.

ANDY'S STORY

Completing 28 days without a drink, for me, was a massive achievement. I had not felt this good in a long time. My head was clear, my body leaner and fitter. My vitality and zest had returned – I felt powerful. Not in a superhero way, but I felt powerful that I had endured the many highs and lows of life booze-free.

It is hard to explain the MASSIVE difference not drinking has made to my life. My relationships thrived and my family adored the new energetic me. I decided to start a degree part-time and also left my job to start a new venture. I was training every day and was at home each evening to kiss the kids goodnight. My life was full and I loved it. My eyes were bright again and everyone I met started to comment on my appearance. I am not saying these things to brag. I am describing the huge difference that quitting alcohol made in my life. I now know for a fact that my life is 10 times

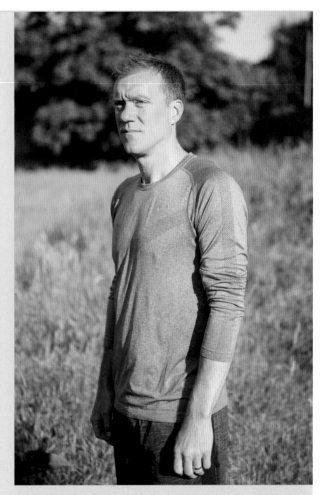

better without the booze. This is a key point I want to make. I only know this because I tried and I kept trying until I cracked it. It was not easy and I slipped up many times on the way. But I dusted myself off, learnt from my mistakes and came back stronger. At the time of writing I am three years alcohol-free and I'm still loving it.

DAY 21

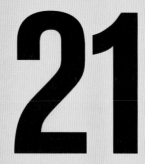

‘NEVER GIVE IN,
NEVER GIVE IN,
NEVER, NEVER,
NEVER, NEVER’
SIR WINSTON CHURCHILL [52]

SURF THE CRAVING URGE

A set of students was asked a simple question, then offered a healthy treat or cake. Those asked to remember a time when they had avoided temptation chose the cake option 70 per cent of the time. Thinking of 'when' reminded them of being 'good', therefore they could be 'bad' now and eat the cake[53].

What's amazing about this study is that the findings were reversed if the students were asked why they had resisted temptation. Asking 'why' rather then 'when' had realigned the students with their overall goals of being healthy, so the cake no longer looked like a reward but a threat to their dreams. The why students then resisted the cake 69 per cent of the time, turning the result on its head.

So if you find yourself in a situation that requires extra willpower, take 10 seconds to remind yourself of all the reasons why you have taken this challenge.

CRAVING

Powerful neurological cravings drive our habits. A great example is our reaction to sugary treats. Our brains learn quickly that under the wrapper there is a tasty delight and it instantly starts to anticipate the sugar.

The world of marketing discovered this a long time ago, and this is why they use branding to let us know exactly what's under the cover and why all fast-food chains look the same.

Cue
Bright-coloured doughnut box.

Routine
Open it, admire the doughnuts and eat them!

Reward
Sugar rush, sweet sensations.

Craving
You are biologically programmed to crave high-carb/sugary foods. On spotting the box, craving starts, the routine is played, the habit loop closes and a habit is formed.

The next time you see the same box in the right context, your brain lights up and starts to crave the sugar rush. You find yourself drawn to the box and then, without really thinking, you find you have opened it and stuffed three pink doughnuts into your mouth. Fifteen minutes later you feel awful as your blood sugar levels come crashing down. You berate yourself for not having the willpower to resist and promise yourself next time will be different.

But now a habit has started to form and the next time you try to resist you will feel disappointed. The brain likes to get its own way and will pursue this even in the face of rational sense. This is a key point: your brain and body are now fighting against you to achieve something you have rationally decided is not good for you. You can't understand why you keep reaching for the cake, the beer, the cigarette – it is not because you are weak-willed, but your evolutionary self has ganged up on you to get what it wants.

The way to overcome these powerful habits is to first notice them. This is why awareness is so important to habit-change and why mindfulness is such a powerful skill to learn. The following exercise will help combat this biological urge.

 RESISTING CRAVINGS

There is plenty of evidence that demonstrates how mindfulness can help people resist cravings[54]. Sarah Bowen is a champion of mindful acceptance. Her work suggests that rather than ignoring cravings we should face them head on, and in doing so we take away their power.

In a study she took two groups of smokers and offered the first group training in mindful acceptance, which she named 'surfing the urge'. The other group received no such training.

The idea behind 'surfing the urge' is that rather than ignoring cravings, the group was told to feel what was going on in their bodies and minds when the cravings struck.

They were encouraged to work with these feelings, to surf these urges safe in the knowledge that, just like a real ocean, these waves of craving would eventually break and wash up on the shore. They were not told to cut back or stop smoking, just to make a note of how many cigarettes they smoked each day and also to note the intensity of the cravings.

At first there was no difference between the two groups. But as the week progressed, the 'surf the urge' group had cut back by a massive 37 per cent, while the control group had shown no change. Also many of the 'surfing the urge' group began to demonstrate that they no longer needed cigarettes as a relief. They felt better equipped to face life's stressors head on, without the crutch of nicotine.

This exercise will work fantastically within this challenge, so let's give it a try.

SURFING THE URGE

The next time you feel a craving to drink, remember this exercise and surf the urge:

1. First acknowledge the fact that you're experiencing a craving. Then, wherever you are, take a few deep breaths. Whether standing or sitting, just feel yourself slow down and relax. Next notice where the craving is presenting itself within your body; what do these sensations feel like and where are they coming from? For example, is the craving coming from your stomach, that then flows up and outwards, trying to propel you to take action and drink…?

2. Now focus on just one specific area where the urge is coming from. Really go deep into these sensations: what do they feel like, what are they encouraging you to do? Don't be afraid to go close to these cravings. Get to know what's really driving you.

3. Repeat this process with each area of craving that you sense. Describe each sensation and how it evolves over time. For example, my lips are tingling in anticipation and I can imagine the taste of alcohol in my mouth. Just notice each time exactly how these urges feel and stay with them.

4. As you sit with this craving, release the tension with every breath. Just imagine that each time you breathe out you are moving towards the end of the craving. Stay with this process until the craving has totally passed and the waves of urges have broken. Lots of people find that after only a few minutes all urges have vanished.

The idea of this exercise is not to make the urges go away, but to experience them in a different light. Rather than trying to ignore them you face up to them. Stare them down and wait until they're gone. By practising this habit breaker you will learn so much more about your cravings and how to smash them.

☑ I AM NOT FEELING THE BENEFITS

Not everyone will experience all the alcohol-free advantages this early in the challenge. There is a tendency to see and read about everyone getting these amazing results and worry about why it's not happening for you. This often leads to frustration and a lack of motivation to continue on this adventure. But please stick with it; the benefits will come, you just need more time. For lots of people the real magic happens between 30 and 90 days, so keep going – the best is yet to come.

So don't worry if you don't feel on top of the world just yet, because you will soon.

WEEK 3 – REFLECTION

WHAT LESSONS HAVE YOU LEARNT?

You now have three weeks alcohol-free under your belt, which is amazing. Before you finish up the week, let's take some time to reflect on the lessons you have learnt during your challenge so far. These lessons could have arisen from a slip-up, a near miss or a friend who was more supportive that you ever imagined.

Through our trials and, often, failures we learn and grow as a person. By reflecting on your challenge there is an opportunity to realise where you have gained strength and wisdom in adversity which will serve you way beyond this adventure.

Take a few minutes now to note down all the lessons you have discovered so far.

Great work! You are well on your way to becoming a 28-day alcohol-free champion.

FILL OUT THE QUICK PROGRESS TRACKER BELOW

Once you fill out this week's tracker, have a look over your previous results and see if you can notice a positive upward trend.

Give yourself a rating out of 10 for each of the following categories, with 1 being a poor rating and 10 being amazing.

Better yet, record your responses so you can track your changes over time at **members.oneyearnobeer.com/Test/Week3.**

QUICK PROGRESS TRACKER	
HAPPINESS	/10
MOTIVATION	/10
PRODUCTIVITY	/10
SLEEP	/10
ENERGY	/10
TIME	/10
EXERCISE	/10
OVERALL SCORE	/70

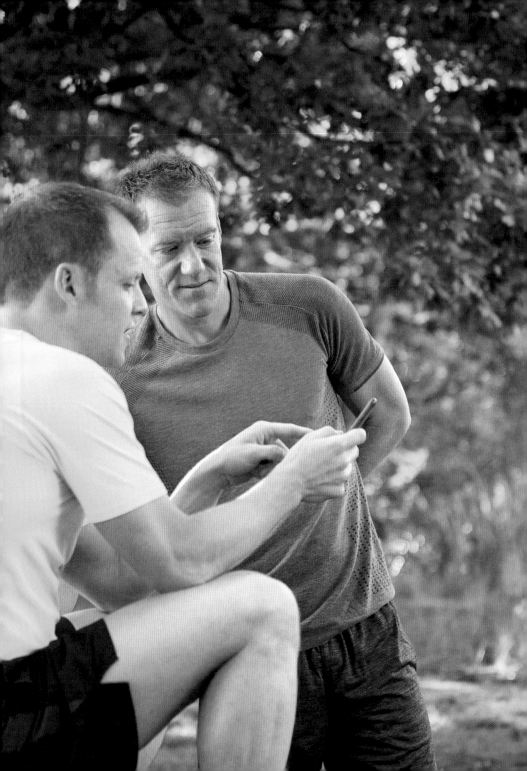

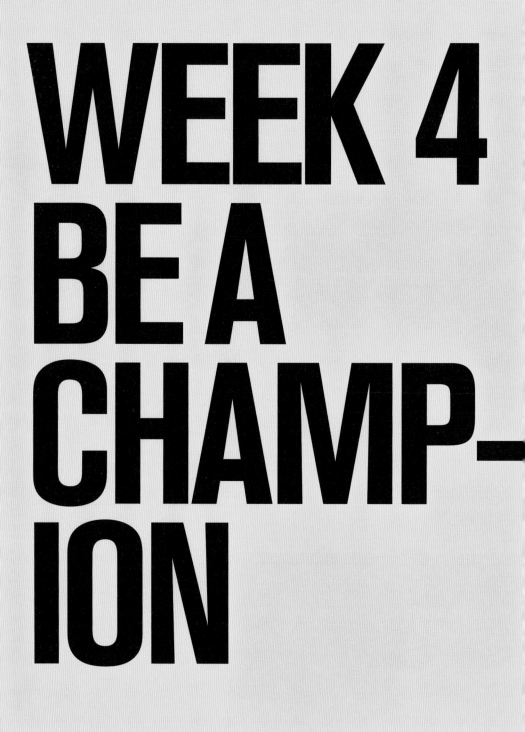

WEEK 4
BE A CHAMP-ION

You now have three weeks under your belt as an alcohol-free Olympian. Wow! We would wager that you are now feeling tip-top. It is often during Week 4 that the alcohol-free advantages start to spiral together to take your well-being to a whole new level. Better sleep provides motivation and energy to exercise. More exercise improves mental well-being, which reduces stress and anxiety. Improved mental health can pave the way to better relationships, more productivity and a rejuvenated social and work life. This spiral keeps going, melding all these factors together, which is why you will hear us say that this challenge is not just about giving up alcohol – it is so much more than that.

In this week you might hear your first 'Wow, you look amazing'. It is very often at this point in the challenge that this starts to happen; friends who have not seen you for a while might notice a difference in your face, body and mentality. This is a great moment and provides the leverage to see you over the finish line and beyond.

This week is also about setting some goals and stretching your willpower muscles to take on those other big life challenges. The skills you are learning will serve you way beyond the 28 days. Having said that, this is not a week to drop your guard, so we have a few ideas to keep you on your toes and ensure you achieve challenge glory.

DAY 22

'LEARN FROM THE MISTAKES OF OTHERS. YOU CAN'T LIVE LONG ENOUGH TO MAKE THEM ALL YOURSELF'

MATTHEW SYED [55]

MODEL YOUR HABITS ON SOMEONE YOU ADMIRE

The Sage was a mythical role model for ancient philosophers. These philosophers tried to emulate this Supreme Being; they understood that they would never quite reach the Sage's level of perfection, but by trying they believed they could find a path to wisdom and the good life.

Although the philosophical Sage can provide wonderful examples of how to live on earth, it helps to have mortal role models, too. These could include people who have overcome adversity or excelled in life. They may have demonstrated tremendous courage or they might simply lead a humble yet virtuous life. They could be a friend, family member, athlete or politician. The key is to value their strengths, not their superficial achievements, such as good looks or wealth.

We find ourselves in a wonderful age when we can harness the power of the internet and books to discover so much about our chosen role models. NLP is a practice developed to help communication and personal development which is based on the idea that we can model success. By uncovering how these great people conducted their lives, how they thought, trained, worked and ate, we can leverage off their experience.

Of course, there are physical limits to this idea, but in trying there are many wonderful lessons to be unearthed. For example, if you wanted extra motivation and guidance on how to love life alcohol-free you might look up to Rich Roll, the alcohol-free wellness guru, as a role model. To take advantage of his knowledge you should get to know what makes him tick. Perhaps read his books, listen to his podcast and discover as much as you can about his journey.

We could all use a little guidance in life. Never underestimate the need to learn from others who have been through the same experiences. If you were about to embark on a trek through an unknown jungle you would find a local guide to lead you safely, someone who had walked the path many times before and succeeded in reaching the destination. It is the same in life; you don't have to tackle uncharted waters yourself, find a guide who has been there before. Learn what they know, how they feel and what mistakes they have made. You will be amazed how much easier your journey becomes when you have someone to show you the way.

Take a few minutes right now to think about someone you admire, who could help you on this alcohol-free challenge or generally in life. Perhaps get to know them a little better, learn what makes them tick and model your world on theirs.

SHE SHOOTS, SHE SCORES!

Part of this habit-change process is to start planning your new healthy world. Now that you have so much extra energy and time, what goals and dreams could you go after?

Take 10 minutes to starting thinking about all the goals you would love to achieve.

Use the headings below as a guide; dream big and don't hold back. Push yourself – you are capable of so much more than you ever believe. Inject a tiny amount of reality, but go for it at the same time.

— **Health goals**
— **Career goals**
— **Relationship goals**
— **Finances and lifestyle goals**
— **Personal goals.**

Enjoy the feelings of dreaming big, but remember the key that unlocks the power of goals is action. So make sure to action one of these goals today – send the email, book the course or make the phone call.

THE VELCRO EFFECT

As soon as you write down your goals, you will find that resources, people and opportunities start to appear as if by magic. This serendipity factor is one of the greatest benefits of goal setting.

Have you ever considered buying a specific type of car, then suddenly you spot them everywhere? It's the same when you set some goals. Once you have made a commitment and written it down, your subconscious mind acts like Velcro, sticking to the things that are needed to achieve these aims. Suddenly you notice the clues that help you on your way, when previously these hidden gems would pass you by. This is why it is so important to get your goals out in the open, to help your mind know what it should focus on.

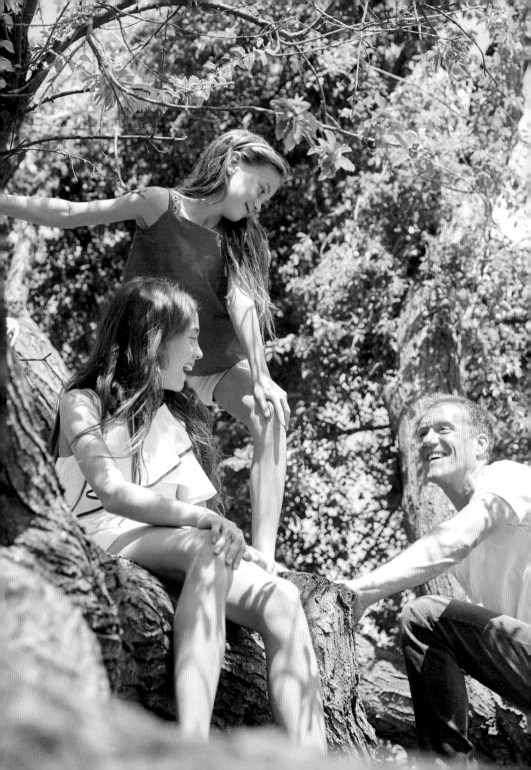

DAY 23

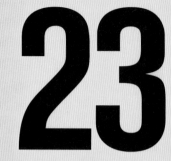

"SPEND YOUR FREE TIME THE WAY YOU LIKE, NOT THE WAY YOU THINK YOU'RE SUPPOSED TO"
SUSAN CAIN [56]

COME HOME TO YOUR BODY

Too many of us have forgotten how to listen to our bodies. The noise of hangovers and lethargy drowns out these internal cries for help. It is too easy at the first sign of a problem to take a pill and write it off. We are a society that has a pill for every ill. This is further confused by a tendency to blame lack of energy, pain, anxiety and stomach upset on booze. In many cases this may be true, but it could be down to something else. What if your body is trying to tell you something? What if it is crying out for help? Maybe your diet is causing you problems. It's hard to hear these cries when hangovers rule.

☑ GET A FULL SERVICE

Now that the cloud of alcohol has lifted, you can hear your body again. Have you recently had a full medical check-up? If not, why not use the cash saved from this challenge for a full service (see Resources, page 216). It's time to treat your body like an athlete's. It is the only one you'll ever have, so you should look after it.

Put a line in the sand of your health, note your statistics and grab this opportunity to improve all your health markers. Perhaps you could lose some weight, lower your cholesterol or reduce your blood pressure?

ANDY'S STORY

In my mid-30s I started to suffer from rosacea, which is a chronic skin complaint that produces the classic whisky drinker's red pimpled cheeks and nose. So I went to the doctor who gave me some pills. They helped a bit, but I still had the occasional outbreak. Here I was taking daily pills for a chronic skin problem and still my skin had not cleared up. I resigned myself to the fact that I would have to live with this uncomfortable problem. I quit alcohol and everything changed.
I would love to say that once I cut out alcohol it vanished. It didn't, but it did get better. What made the real difference was that once the hangovers were out of the way I had the time, energy and cleaner life to evaluate my dietary choices. Slowly I adjusted my diet from your basic meat-eating salad-dodging to vegetarian, which evolved into the wholefood, plant-based diet it is today. And guess what? No more rosacea. By quitting alcohol and changing my diet I have stopped this chronic problem in its tracks.

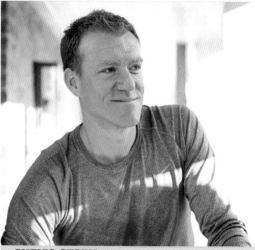

THINK LONG TERM

Studies have shown that thinking about our long-term goals can have a positive influence on our behaviour in the present[57]. When we forget our long-term goals we are more vulnerable to cravings and slip-ups.

LONG-TERM GOALS

Think of the last time you fell off the wagon. What was the reason? Imagine this situation in your mind: try to remember where you were and who you were with. Were you feeling pressured or relaxed? Build up a detailed mental picture of your temptation.

Now take a couple of minutes to reflect on how this short-term thinking slip-up affected your long-term aims. Then try this exercise:

Imagine yourself in the scenario above, faced with the drink of your choice – only you're prepared. Before you react, think of your long-term goals. Imagine how strong and confident you will feel for exerting self-control. Do you look better, feel better and perform better? Own these feelings – you have achieved so much.

Now imagine yourself making the right choice, showing the courage of your convictions. Imagine turning down the drink and how good it feels to stay on track and how empowered you are for not giving in.

When you face temptation, take a deep breath, think of your long-term goals and make the choice that's right for you.

ANDY'S STORY

Of course, I am totally biased, but I have enjoyed every part of my alcohol-free challenge. One of the greatest findings, on a personal level, was discovering that I'm an introvert. Had you asked me the introvert/extrovert question at any point up until recently I would have replied with confidence: 'extrovert'.

Many of my former social activities lost their allure once alcohol was removed. Large gatherings and busy places held less appeal. I started to find happiness in words, education, nature, family, food and the simple things in life. I had a real sense that I was changing, but on reflection I was not changing – just reverting to the real me.

Around this time I picked up a wonderful book called Quiet *by Susan Cain, which blew my mind. Cain describes how extroversion is prized in our modern world, but there is real power* in being an introvert. As I read each page I came to the startling conclusion that I was, and always had been, an introvert.

Full of excitement, I called my wife and said 'You know what I am?' After a long pause, in which I am sure she was thinking 'A ginger fool? The worst putter-outer of garbage in the world?', I declared, 'I'm an introvert!'

She cracked up laughing. I think my presentation was somewhat over the top, but we both agreed that I am without doubt an introvert. This made so much sense. I had been pretending to be something I wasn't for most of my adult life. Alcohol was my gateway to extroversion.

One of the great internal struggles I had regularly faced was how my character was so different the day after a night out. It was confusing being the life and soul of the party, the larger-than-life guy one minute, only to feel an overwhelming desire to shy away from that person the next.

We all have friends who are genuinely the life and soul, whether in or out of the bar setting. They are just as gregarious the morning after, because this is who they truly are. They are the same character with or without alcohol. I was shy in social settings, I find small talk hard and being social for social's sake exhausting. I can fly like a social butterfly when required to, but it zaps my energy. Even though I have discovered

> **❝ I HAD BEEN PRETENDING TO BE SOMETHING I WASN'T FOR MOST OF MY ADULT LIFE. ALCOHOL WAS MY GATEWAY TO EXTROVERSION. ❞**

this person was not the real me, letting go of this identity was the hardest part of giving up alcohol – while at the same time the most rewarding. Not having to be that guy any more was a breath of fresh air. I am now confident enough to say 'no' to certain events, knowing that they will drain my energy.

My guess is that many people use alcohol as a gateway to extroversion and to overcome social shyness. I totally get this, but it's tiring and fraught with disappointment. The internal conflict this creates is not worth the effort, and the only way to keep up this pretence is to keep drinking.

Let's be real about this – we all know that alcohol provides a fake confidence for a short space of time, but let's also agree that it quickly melts the following day, to be replaced by anxiety and lethargy. Living like this drains our energy, while being true to ourselves fills us with life and vitality. Finding your true self is tough, especially when it runs contrary to what you have believed for many years. Hopefully this story will encourage those who feel like this to make the effort because being your true self is one of life's great joys.

DAY 24

‘ KINDNESS IN WORDS CREATES CONFIDENCE. KINDNESS IN THINKING CREATES PROFOUNDNESS. KINDNESS IN GIVING CREATES LOVE ’

LAO TZU [58]

CHOOSE TO BE HAPPY RIGHT NOW

**Before you think we have gone all Tony Robbins on you, there is
something really powerful about a life without booze. It's strange,
but you will, over time, build massive strength as you face life's
challenges without the crutch of alcohol. We are not just talking about
the obvious social situations, but life situations, too. Those stressful
moments that you previously tried to cover up with alcohol can now
be faced with a clear head. Over time you will encounter many of
these situations, and as the bumper sticker says: sh*t happens.
Going alcohol-free will not prevent life's problems, but for perhaps
the first time in a long while you will face these obstacles fully armed
with all your senses.**

We guarantee that once you have overcome
a few of these 'tests' without reverting to old
patterns you will emerge a much stronger
person. You will wake up one day feeling
really powerful. It's hard to explain, but there
is real strength in knowing you can deal
with all that life has to throw at you, without
alcohol. As the days progress and you
conquer both social and life challenges you
will start to feel a real power within.

I'LL BE HAPPY WHEN ...

The worst phrase in the English language:
'I'll be happy when I have [fill in blank]',
or 'I'll be happy when I don't have
[fill in blank]'.

Why wait? Why wait until you have the
money, the bigger car, the better body?
Why wait until you don't have the mortgage,
the dead-end job, the illness?

WHY NOT BE HAPPY AND CONTENT RIGHT NOW?

Avoid turning your challenge experience
into 'I'll be happy when I get through two
weeks, or reach the end.' Right now, right
this second when you have stopped drinking
and begun to change your life, the past has
gone and the future is not decided. Right
now you have succeeded in every way. In this
very moment you are trying something new
that empowers you.

Once you are content in this very
moment, the rest comes easily. You will
achieve your goals and enjoy every step of
the journey to reach them. And if you don't?
You can refine your goals and start again, safe
in the knowledge that they are a guide and
not the end destination to your well-being.

MOTION IS EMOTION

There is an old saying, 'motion is emotion' – and it's true, your mind and body are one. When both are aligned you are at your most powerful. This is essentially the message behind this challenge: to create the ultimate healthy lifestyle that you need in order to have your mind and body working as one.

Our mental state is affected by our internal thoughts and our physiology. The exercise below is a wonderful hack to hijack your body and change your mental state.

STATE MATE

If you are feeling stressed after a long day your mental and physical state might be wound up tight. It is in these unhelpful states that wrong choices are often made.

We totally understand that a quick way to change state is through alcohol – we are not denying this, but there is always an emotional and physical price to pay for this solution. So rather than take the easy route and derail your challenge, here is a great exercise from the world of NLP that will help you shift to a resourceful state in an instant.

Take 20 seconds to perform the following exercise. You will feel a difference in your physical state, which will trigger a change in your mental state so that you become bright and alert:

1. Starting position: sitting or standing, with your shoulders bent inwards towards your chest and your back curved downwards.

Let your arms and hands swing down by your sides. Lower your head in line with your shoulders. Basically, you are going for the sulky teenager posture.

Note how you feel in this position – we wager you don't feel dynamic ...

2. Now gradually uncurl from this position. Bring your shoulders back slowly.

3. Start to raise your head. Straighten the spine and neck to create a nice straight line from the top of the head to the bottom of the spine.

4. Pull your shoulders back, let your arms relax, make sure your head is upright and looking forward.

If you are sitting down, stand up.

Take a nice full breath as you stand tall.

This posture is bright and alert.

Note how you feel and now make the choice that is right for you.

This is a wonderful demonstration of how the mind and body are intrinsically linked. The next time you feel unmotivated, overwhelmed or stressed, try this exercise – you will snap from an unhelpful state into a resourceful state, which paves the way for choosing to take the right actions.

RANDOM ACTS OF KINDNESS

Science has now shown, which most of us instinctively know, that random acts of kindness – no matter how big or small – have a huge positive impact on our well-being[59]. What's more, the beneficiary of this kindness also receives a well-being lift.

You might ask what has this got to do with giving up alcohol? Our answer is: everything. The brighter your alcohol-free world, the more motivation you will have to stay on this path. This is such a beautiful idea, so why not just give it a go?

Today, keep an eye out for an opportunity to perform at least one random act of kindness. This could be for a family member, partner, friend or a complete stranger – the effect is the same.

It could be as simple as holding open a door, paying a compliment or giving up your seat on the train. The key is to do it, no questions asked.

These acts can produce kindness contagion, which cause more and more kindness, whether applied to family or strangers. A fantastic pay it forward effect, where your kind deeds are replicated time and time again, spreading outward. What a brilliant exercise!

Over time you will start to notice more and more opportunities to offer some extra kindness, creating an upward spiral of giving.

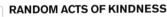

RANDOM ACTS OF KINDNESS – NO MATTER HOW BIG OR SMALL – HAVE A HUGE POSITIVE IMPACT ON OUR WELL-BEING.

DAY 25

'IMPRESSING PEOPLE IS UTTERLY DIFFERENT FROM BEING TRULY IMPRESSIVE'

RYAN HOLIDAY [60]

LEAD BY EXAMPLE

Other people's goals, both good and bad, can influence our worlds, so it is important to protect ourselves from negative influences. If you can, imagine that you're building your own well-being armour through which no emotional junk or limiting beliefs will penetrate. To help strengthen this armour, remind yourself of your goals at the start of every day. Stick a note on the mirror or create one on your smartphone. This process of reminding yourself every day of your aims will help protect you against the negative influence of others.

As your day progresses and you notice other people slipping – eating cake, getting stressed or drinking alcohol – be confident that you are strong and staying true to your goals. Use these feelings of strength to make you more determined to stay on track.

☑ LEAD BY EXAMPLE – THE ULTIMATE MOTIVATOR

Science has shown that our habits are contagious[61]. This has to be one of the most powerful reasons to follow your dreams. Your behaviour affects those you love and care for. Once you start to thrive, your loved ones will pick up on these traits and their chances of flourishing will increase, too. If you lose weight, control your temper, get fit, learn to relax or quit drinking, all these habits might flow to those around you. Live by example and your children, family and friends will benefit. For parents, brothers, sisters and partners, this has to be the ultimate motivator. We all want our loved ones to be happy and healthy. It is amazing to discover that cultivating healthy living in

your own life will also give those close to you the best shot at improving their health and happiness.

Draw strength and motivation from knowing that every step you take on your challenge will have a positive effect on those you love.

DOES MY BUM LOOK BIG IN THESE GENES?

We have all heard the classic excuse as to why people behave the way they do:

'It's down to the genes: my dad had a temper; mum is overweight; high blood pressure runs in the family; my old man was a drinker ...'

Or:

'I may as well accept it, the size of my bum is down to my mum – you can't fight your genes ...'

Let's clear this up straight away for all those people who like to use genes as an excuse not to try. The science of genetics is rapidly advancing and, like most sciences, opinions are starting to change. Genes are no longer viewed as fixed traits[62], but biases that can be switched on and off depending on lifestyle and environmental factors. Just because your dad's a grouch or your mother is overweight, it doesn't mean you have to be. Of course, you might be slightly predisposed to pessimism or your mother's fuller figure, but as we have discovered many times, you are capable of unbelievable change – genetics are only a small part of the story. Using your genes as an excuse not to try to change for the better is not an 'excuse'. If you can change the shape of your brain through meditation you can learn to look on the bright side.

It is the same with drinking. Perhaps someone in your family is a drinker and perhaps you've been told it's in your genes. Well, you are proving this theory wrong. Take massive confidence from this fact, that those supposed genetic theories are just that – theories.

Grab this encouragement and challenge all those genes that might be holding you back. Don't stop with alcohol; you have the power to change tempers, waistlines, how you act and the way you feel.

GET READY FOR THE 'WOWS'

As you move towards the end of Week 4 you will start to look and feel great. Get ready to see an old friend or colleague who produces your first 'Wow, you look amazing!' This is a wonderful feeling and one that makes it worth the effort. Take huge confidence and pride from your achievements. Your life is changing and improving every day.

A word of caution: be sure to stay on track and keep yourself in check. You would not want to get overconfident and drop your guard now. Take a deep breath when faced with a random situation that would normally spark a drinking session. Remember the ambush and be prepared for a scenario that crops up out of the blue. Take a quick 60-second pause – think of your long-term goals, your family and your health, then make the right choice. Or perhaps go for a walk, or a drive or sit and listen to some music. Find some space to relax away from the tempting situation.

Congratulations on your first 'wow'!

LIFE IS ONE MASSIVE SELF-FULFILLING PROPHECY

'Whether you think you can, or you think you can't – you're right!'

This great quote from Henry Ford (see Day 15) says it all. Life is one giant self-fulfilling prophecy. For those of us who look on the bright side, guess what? We seem to find the best in most situations. Others who believe they will fail very often manage to prove themselves right.

As you have discovered during your challenge, you can change your beliefs, even long-held ones. You can also choose the things you want to believe in, which will steer your life in that direction.

Don't settle for hand-me-down beliefs and don't be afraid to challenge and change any beliefs that are holding you back. Build the world that you want. If you have a big challenge ahead, put your mind and body into it. Build your belief that you can achieve the dream and then reap the rewards.

FOREST BATHING

Oh no, we hear you cry, now they want us to take a bath outdoors! Well, not quite. But we do want you to find a green space. Once again, the scientists have confirmed what we instinctively know: that time spent in nature is good for us[63].

The Japanese have been wise to the healing power of nature for millennia but they have only recently coined the phrase 'Shinrin-yokko', which translates as 'forest bathing.' There is a bundle of research that demonstrates the power of nature to improve our well-being. To be clear, this does not have to mean a hike in the forest – even a small amount of green can make a big difference. Keeping houseplants in your living room or getting views of nature

from a window can be enough to stimulate these benefits.

Patients recover quicker from surgery when they have a view of nature outside, while office workers who have plants within view experience reduced fatigue, anger, anxiety and depression. Studies also reveal that being outdoors in nature improves immune systems and increases the number of anti-cancer proteins. We are particularly interested in this forest bathing because it improves our willpower friend, heart-rate variability, which provides those extra gears to deal with cravings.

So not only is spending time outdoors a beautiful experience, it also offers myriad well-being benefits and will be invaluable on this challenge.

GO GREEN EXERCISE

Today and every day, where possible aim to spend some time bathing in nature. This does not have to be a national park, it could be an oasis of green in a major city. The idea is to immerse yourself for as long as you can – even just 5–10 minutes on a lunch break – so that you can breathe deep and wallow in nature's goodness. When you open your eyes to green spaces you will find them everywhere, even in the busiest of cities. So there is no reason why you cannot find time for forest bathing every day.

DAY 26

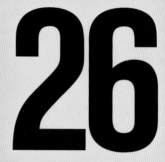

‘THINGS DO NOT CHANGE; WE CHANGE’
HENRY DAVID THOREAU [64]

RUARI'S STORY OF FULL CONTROL

At this point on your adventure you might be considering returning to drinking, so we've put together a little framework to help you resist the temptation. If you are set on continuing this challenge or considering not drinking again, we urge you to read on. There are some valid points here, especially regarding boundaries, that you may want to pay attention to.

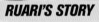

RUARI'S STORY

When I chose to stop drinking I didn't do it with the goal of never drinking again – I chose to stop drinking for a set period, 90 days. It was during those 90 days that I realised how brilliant I felt and how much my life had changed. My relationships, my focus, my energy, my passion were all back to their best. I had been hiding behind a social glass of fuzz. Brain fuzz.

I did a year with pretty much nothing; I tasted a few wines at dinners before it was served to my table, I went to a whisky tasting and over the course of an evening probably drank a single shot in different tastes – talk about into the lion's den. But all in all I was alcohol-free for a year. I then decided to try a drink now and again, which led up to Christmas Day – a few days in a row drinking a little and then binge drinking on the day itself led to a huge fallout between my wife and I. I knew the common denominator was booze, so I removed it again. I then took on almost another year, but on a couple of occasions I had a drink. A pint here and a whisky there, perhaps on three or four occasions. I still wasn't done testing. There were feelings inside of being trapped by something externally controlling me. You see, I've always had a problem with being controlled. Now I felt trapped by OYNB expecting me to be alcohol-free and my freedom to choose. Interesting conundrum. So I needed to see where this led me and I decided to have a drink now and again.

I knew I wasn't going to be on a slippery slope because I felt in control. Over Christmas with

DRINKING: THE REALITIES

There are, without doubt, some occasions when you feel at a disadvantage without a drink. We're not saying these moments don't exist, they do! However, they are far, far fewer than you think. There is a tendency to believe that having a drink, or several, with a potential in-law or new client makes a big difference. We promise you could have taken on these occasions without drinking and been just as successful – if not even more so.

The thing is, let's not pretend that one drink needs to be 20, or that you need to do two nights in a row, or carry on for an extra three hours, etc. etc. The vast majority of our drinking is habit.

So if you can follow a simple framework – and this will be unique to everyone – it will help guide you back into drinking with control. Some people call it mindful drinking; we want to call it full control.

WHY MODERATION IS SO TRICKY

I think the concept of managing your drinks on a daily or weekly level is incredibly hard. Sure, it works for some people, and those people probably know who they are already before they try it because they moderate in many other areas of life. They can take it or leave it.

I think the best way to go back to drinking is to constantly evaluate what's going on for you and to make an assessment based on that moment. There are reasons why you might choose to drink, and reasons why you should choose not to. They will be individual, but these ideas might get you started.

Times you might consider drinking:

— **Big events, moments, celebrations**
— **One-off business event that will lead to something positive**
— **When you feel like it.**

Reasons you should avoid drinking:

— **Stressed, worried, anxious; feel you need a drink**
— **Pressure from others to drink – either before the event or during it.**

OVERALL ASSESSMENT
Did I feel the need to change my relationship with alcohol before this challenge?

☐ Yes – depending on how intimate this reason is, consider extending your challenge beyond 28 days.

☐ No – you have it under control already, what are you worried about?

Have you been to many high-pressure events and enjoyed them alcohol-free; have you realised the next day you didn't need booze?

☐ Yes, a couple of times.

☐ Yes, on many occasions. I love it!

☐ No.

DRINKING HABITS
Could you start a drink now and leave it halfway? Well, when you see it for what it is, you will be able to, or just choose not to have it, full stop.

☐ Does one always lead to another? Addictive behaviour can be hard to control, so perhaps increase your distance first.

☐ Do you feel pressure to drink from others that you find hard to ignore? You haven't learnt enough yet; more awareness is needed; it's all false.

☐ Do you feel you are the type of person who will go off the rails if you start drinking again? (Why risk it? There's no up side!)

BOUNDARIES
Once you make the decision to drink again, if you cross these boundaries consider another alcohol-free challenge. Perhaps a longer one this time: 90 or even 365 days.

— **Drunk, slurring words, generally past the point of control**
— **Angry/shouting/snappy/irritable/ bad mood after drinking**
— **Hangovers twice in a month**
— **Skipping exercise or personal training because of drinking**
— **Once you have one, you need another and another ...**
— **Find yourself filling your glass more than others.**

Alcohol is sneaky; you've been associating it with good times since you can remember good times! For more resources go to www.oneyearnobeer.com/book-resources.

DAY 27

‹WHAT YOU
DO EVERY DAY
MATTERS MORE
THAN WHAT
YOU DO ONCE
IN A WHILE›
GRETCHEN RUBIN [65]

THE BIG TEST THAT'S JUST AROUND THE CORNER

Hopefully by now you're fully aligned with your goal of staying alcohol-free, for the next two days, if not longer, but don't underestimate its pull – you have probably spent a large chunk of your life physically and mentally conditioning yourself to drink. These habitual pathways still exist; you have simply changed them to new, healthy, empowering routines.

These bad habitual patterns can hang around for a while and are ready and waiting to pounce, given half a chance. So make sure you prepare for your big events. Know exactly what you are going to say and what you are going to drink. Be ready when you walk into the reception and the waiter shoves a glass of champagne into your hand. Be ready to gently hand it back in exchange for an orange juice or give it to your partner or a friend. Get through the first hour and you will fly through the rest of the occasion. It will be full of 'Wows' and 'You look great'. People will want to know your story and as the day progresses you will find many people confessing that they wish they could take a break from booze, too.

Best of all – and do remember this – when you wake the next day feeling like the hero you are, take five seconds to pat yourself on the back for having made this amazing change. While you are up and around enjoying all life has to offer, all the boozers will still be in bed, in bits.

 THE BEER BACKPACK
You are so close to your milestone of 28 days alcohol-free. But there might still be a long way to go before you completely change your relationship with alcohol forever.

Here is an exercise to help you on the last part of this alcohol-free adventure.

Start with a few deep breaths, wherever you are. Then find a position that you can stay relaxed in for the next five minutes. There are no rights or wrongs here, just do whatever feels right.

Close your eyes if you prefer and imagine the following scenario: you are on a climbing expedition and you find yourself on the way to camp. You have already climbed a large section of mountain to reach this point and just over the ridge is your destination. The tents are warm, the fires are lit and the food is on. This last push will take you to the first big milestone. Initial challenge complete.

Now imagine your backpack is full of a heavy load, consisting of all the past negatives that drinking brought with it. The sort of issues that weighed you down both mentally and physically, making life one long slog.

Perhaps your pack contains:

— **Fake courage**
— **Stress and anxiety**
— **Lethargy**
— **Lack of motivation**
— **Lost time**
— **Unhealthy food**
— **Poor fitness.**

Perhaps your pack is old because of all the money you wasted on alcohol?

Take some time to really imagine how hard the climb to base camp will be carrying this heavy load. We wager you feel physically tired at this point.

Now imagine taking a deep breath and emptying all these heavy negatives onto the snow. Watch them as they slowly sink away.

Now gently imagine re-packing your bag with all the positives you have experienced during the challenge so far.

Perhaps you might add:

— **The time you have won back**
— **Extra energy**
— **Rush of motivation**
— **Vitality**
— **Exercise routines**
— **Better diet.**

You can even use a brand-new bag bought from all the money you have saved.

Build this picture bright in your mind. What can you feel, smell, taste and sense as you lift this lighter load onto your back, ready to make the last push home?

Imagine yourself making this journey effortlessly towards base camp to complete step one of your challenge. How good does this feel? How proud are your loved ones? How do you look? How much confidence does this bring?

Finally, as you experience these wonderful sensations, ask yourself: do I want to continue with this adventure?

 ANDY'S SOBER DANCING CHALLENGE

It's important to realise that we are shaped by our social cultures. Drinking was a huge part of mine; sober dancing was not. Nor is it now. Ask your average male over the age of 13 to dance sober in public and they'll probably ask you to shoot them. Just the thought of it is enough to bring most of us out in a cold sweat.

This thought challenged me. Here we are, trying to bring awareness to the fact that we don't need alcohol in our lives, yet the thought of sober dancing turned my stomach. There is light at the end of the tunnel, though, but before we get there, let me share a personal experience.

I was a week into my NLP master practitioner course when all my worst fears were confirmed. There were 50 of us on the course and the threat of something really embarrassing was looming. Suddenly, there was music in the room. I started to panic.

Although nothing was said, or even hinted at, the music was enough to send my mind into overdrive. All I could think was, 'If they make us dance, I'm out of here.'

As the crowd began to notice the music, some of the 'out there' mob started to move. I was instantly jealous of their beautiful carefree spirits, enjoying the moment while I was standing there white with fear. The next thing I knew – and it's a bit of blur! – our tutor, the legendary John Grinder, stepped up to the mic and explained that we were going to have a little fun. 'Shit,' I thought, 'This sounds ominous.'

'What I would like you all to do is free-form dance.'

Is he for real? What has this got to do with NLP? My worst nightmare had come true. I knew I shouldn't have taken this course. I loved these ideas, but this was a step too far for a ginger. I always go bright red at the slightest embarrassment, and at that moment you could have cooked eggs on my forehead. I looked for the exit and my escape. I prayed the ground would open up and swallow me whole. Anything but dance, please, please …

Almost instantly, the 'out there' crew were rocking, arms and legs everywhere. Off they went, enjoying the beat, revelling in the music, smiling, laughing. I was bright red and frozen to the spot. I had no choice but to move in some form, so slowly I lifted an arm, which seemed to weigh a ton. My legs

were like lead as I dragged them from the floor. I moved like someone who had been magnetised trying to haul their body along a fridge door. After five minutes of utter pain, it was over. The music stopped. I was still alive – just.

Once I calmed down and returned to my normal state, the truth was revealed. The whole exercise had been very deliberately designed to scare the life out of us. The idea was to notice how a simple request could change your whole being, both mental and physical. It was one of the most powerful lessons I have been taught, and something that will stay with me forever.

When the original request was made, I was almost angry, because I had wrongly assumed it was just a pointless icebreaker. Now I realised a deeper message lay behind it.

On reflection, I found it fascinating that my perceptions of how society would expect me to behave could have physically stopped my body moving. Here I was, an ex-professional athlete, with total control of my body, feeling unable to move for fear of looking silly.

I still don't relish the idea of sober dancing, but I understand that a mental process caused my pain. I have since danced a few times sober, and while it's still a shocker, it can be sort of fun. For me, it was the last bastion to fall. My life without booze was now complete.

For myself, and probably a lot of you, sober dancing is the ultimate challenge.

But if you can do this, you can do anything. Enjoy the music, have fun and know that you are now unstoppable. Your confidence is back. Cut the rug, moonwalk out of the office – unleash the sober dancer within.

☑ AMBASSADOR

At this stage you know better than anyone how to get through those early weeks and how much brighter your life will be at the end of it, so perhaps you could give something back?

Acts of kindness are good for you, so why not spread some love to those people who are at the start of their alcohol-free journey?

Giving back is such an important part of your challenge experience. You could give some advice to a friend, or log into the OYNB groups online and share your story to inspire others.

Get stuck in and pass it forward. We promise this will make your challenge experience extra special.

TRY NOT TO DROP THE GOOD HABITS

Goals are great for building empowering habits, but all too often, once the goal is reached, the good habits are forgotten. Training for a marathon is a classic example. So many people put themselves through an amazing process of transformation to reach their goal of running 26 miles. They finish the race – and then what? Often they take a well-deserved break and do nothing. The wonderful routines they built up slip away; they no longer have something to aim for so old habits take over and they stop running. This is the equivalent of yo-yo dieting. We go all out to achieve a level of fitness or weight, and then, once it is reached, we let it all go.

There is no point working hard to develop the habits required to take a break from alcohol and then, on reaching the finish line, letting this hard work slip. So watch your drinking habits closely and if old habits rear their head, come back and start the challenge afresh until your healthy habits are so ingrained that total and full control will last you a lifetime.

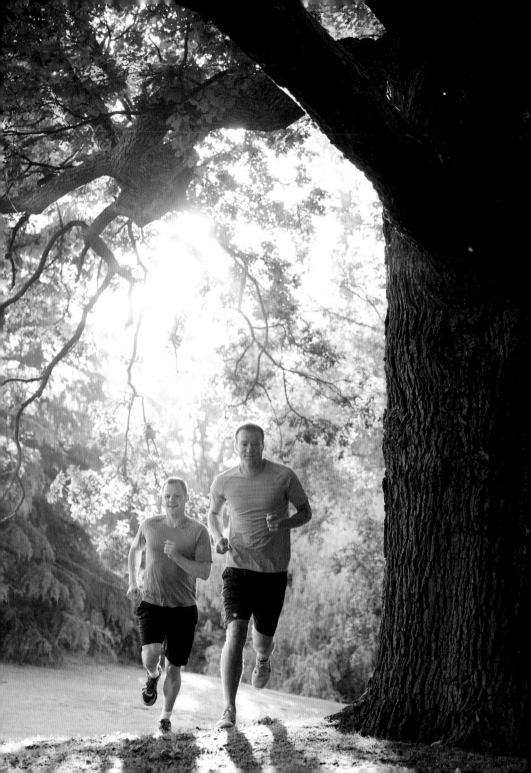

DAY 28

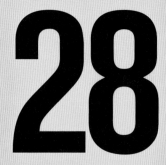

'YOU ARE
A CHAMPION
MY FRIEND'
ANDY AND RUARI

CHAMPION

YOU CHAMPION! 28 DAYS ALCOHOL-FREE!

Perhaps this is the longest break you've had from alcohol since your teens?

We're so proud of you and this is a massive alcohol-free barrier to smash. So enjoy today, revel in the warm feelings this achievement brings. Walk tall and feel proud of how far you have come.

Perhaps take a few minutes to consider your journey so far. What have you learnt, what have you overcome and what has made this challenge extra special?

Write down these feelings on a piece of paper and savour the great feelings this creates, you champion.

Complete your last quick progress tracker below, then look over all your results and see for yourself how far you have progressed.

Give yourself a rating out of 10 for each of the categories, with 1 being a poor rating and 10 being amazing.

Better yet, record your responses so you can track your changes over time at **members.oneyearnobeer.com/Test/Week4.**

Finally, don't forget to take the quick online well-being survey, oneyearnobeer.com/finish-survey, to record your results.

Before you get too comfortable, though, let's talk about your next adventure.

QUICK PROGRESS TRACKER	
HAPPINESS	/10
MOTIVATION	/10
PRODUCTIVITY	/10
SLEEP	/10
ENERGY	/10
TIME	/10
EXERCISE	/10
OVERALL SCORE:	/70

THE HERO'S JOURNEY

Joseph Campbell's wonderful book *The Hero of a Thousand Faces* first introduced to us the timeless concept of the hero's journey. Campbell unearthed a universal truth that all great stories share a single pattern, which he calls the hero's journey. This is essentially a metaphor for our own worldly struggles and triumphs.

Firstly, there is a call to action that takes the hero away from the comfort of their home or present situation. This is followed by an adventure that tests the hero to the limit. The hero faces their worst fears – even potentially death – but overcomes these challenges to rise a stronger person. Changed, they return home with a gift: the story of their adventure. But this is not the end; now enlightened, they are called to more adventures and the cycle continues, as it does in our daily lives. This pattern is found in the great works from the *Odyssey* to religious texts and to more modern tales such as *Star Wars* and *Harry Potter*. It is always the same.

This universal truth fits perfectly with your alcohol-free challenge. There is a calling, a point reached when something has to change. This is followed by a sense that there is more to life outside the comfort zone. By saying yes to this 28-day adventure you have taken yourself away from the norm. You have stepped outside into an unknown world full of tests and trials. There is perhaps a sense of leaving one world and entering another.

You may have faced many demons, trials and worst fears, but by overcoming these obstacles you are growing stronger with each victory. Now the first victory is won, you return wiser, stronger, more confident and with a gift: your story of how you survived and thrived during this 28-day alcohol-free challenge.

But behind the mountains are more mountains and very soon you will have to answer the call of another challenge. We have established that for the majority of people the real magic in this challenge is somewhere between 28 and 80 days – it all depends on the individual. Some people go through a particular slump at around 28 days and this can be a sign that you need to carry on. The magic is just round the corner. We have condensed our challenge to 28 days, and while that is enough for you to get a great insight into the benefits of alcohol-free living, the real changes are just over the horizon.

So if you are now wondering whether to continue, the answer is most definitely YES. Whatever your decision – whether you go back to drinking in full control occasionally, stop completely, or continue with your alcohol-free adventure for another month or two – the choice, as always, is yours.

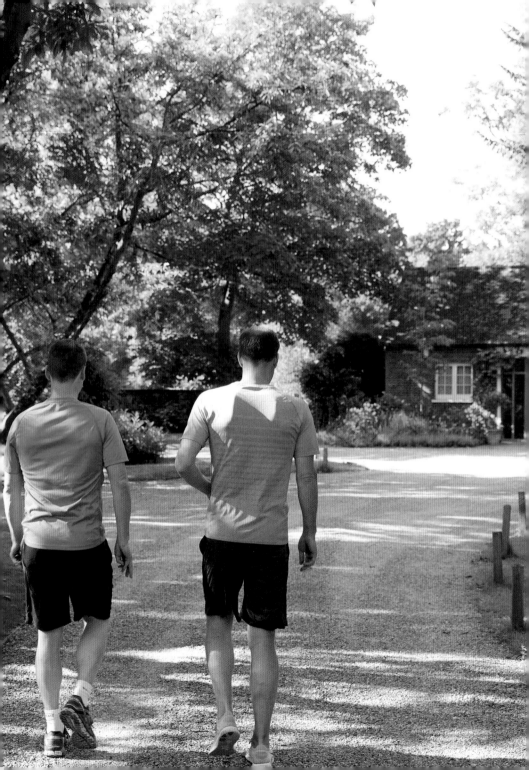

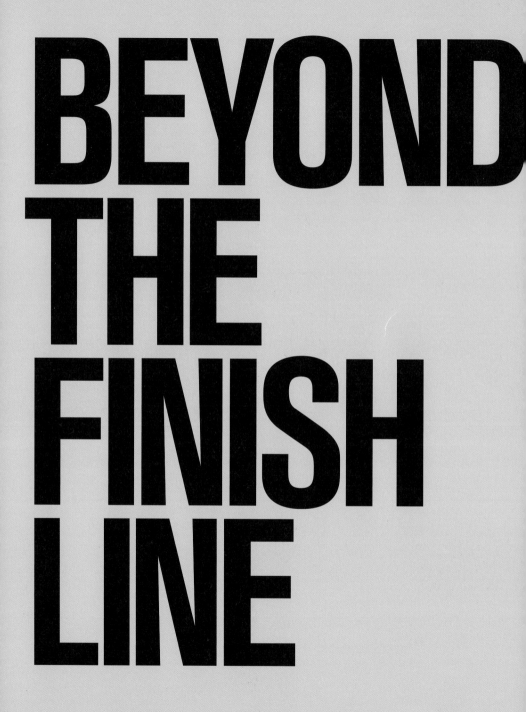

BEYOND THE FINISH LINE

SO WHAT NEXT?

CELEBRATE WITH A DRINK

Of course, this is up to you, but ask yourself, do you want to slip straight back into old habits and feel like death in the morning? And if you continue to 90 days we can (almost) guarantee you'll be thanking us for encouraging you to do so!

CONTINUE WITH THE CHALLENGE

Just imagine how great you will feel after 90 days booze-free. For the vast majority of our OYNB members, the real magic is somewhere around 60–90 days, which is why we so prominently focus on the 90-day challenge. The real fruits of this challenge are ahead of you, so why not head over to www.oneyearnobeer.com and join us?

GO BACK TO DRINKING EVERY NOW AND THEN IN FULL CONTROL

At this stage you might already feel that you have regained full control – and that's amazing. It is worth re-reading the 'The Slip-up' section on page 74 to make sure you stay on track. If you feel yourself slipping, come back and start the challenge again. There is no limit to how many times you take this challenge. We have witnessed thousands of members come back again and again to take another, often longer, challenge. Once a member, always a member, and we are here to support you forever.

FOR THAT REASON, I AM OUT

You may have now reached the conclusion that you're going to stay alcohol-free forever. Life is so rich without alcohol, why bother going back? This proactive life stance will help inspire so many other people to do the same. Congratulations.

WHATEVER YOU DECIDE, PLEASE TRY TO INSPIRE OTHERS

Having completed the challenge, whatever its outcome, you now have the gift of a story to tell, so please help to inspire others to try this challenge. But for now, enjoy being the 28 day alcohol-free champion you are. Massive congratulations.

Andy and Ruari

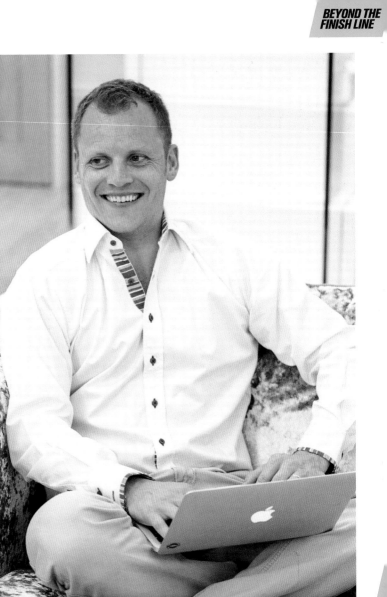

YOUR ADVANTAGE

Before you get started on your long-term alcohol-free adventure, let's do something that almost no other book, website or well-meaning friend ever does when it comes to alcohol. Let's talk about all the amazing advantages that flow your way when you stop drinking.

With years of alcohol-free experience under our belts, along with thousands of inspiring stories from our members, we can now confidently say that if you want to gain a clear advantage in almost every aspect of life, going AF will give you the edge. In the chapter that follows, we have attempted to summarise some of the main advantages that we've discovered over the last few years. This is far from an exhaustive list as the real advantages flow well beyond this selection, but hopefully it's enough to get the message across: going alcohol-free provides you with a massive advantage.

WE KNOW ALL ABOUT THOSE WARM FUZZY FEELINGS

Before we get started, let's inject some realism into what follows. We have been there, seen it, done it and bought the t-shirt when it comes to alcohol. We can't pretend that we haven't had some good times while drinking, so the advantages that follow are not an attempt to divert your attention from those perceived upsides of drinking, because we totally get all the upsides that alcohol

Yet another little thing to reduce stress and give back chill time to my life. With all the money I'm saving on booze I have got myself a cleaner.

KIRSTAN

pretends to offer. We fully accept that alcohol can act as a wonderful state-changing tool, bringing you to a place of relaxation and helping troubles vanish quickly. We also know first-hand that alcohol creates a social lubricant that's hard to beat.

We are not denying any of these things, but none of these perceived upsides comes for free. There is always an emotional and physical price to pay for drinking, and it gets more and more expensive over time. The real problem is that most people start drinking in their teens and never stop, so they forget what it's really like to be alcohol-free. They forget how much more energy, vitality, confidence, motivation and time they had before alcohol was on the scene. It's not until they get a break that they realise just what they were missing and how much alcohol was holding them back.

So our aim is to expose these real costs – not by banging you over the head with the obvious health and social issues, but by showing you all the wonderful benefits that flow your way when you take a break.

DON'T BELIEVE US JUST BECAUSE WE SAY SO

You don't have to take our word for it just because we have years of alcohol-free knowledge. You don't have to believe the doctors, scientists and all-round well-being gurus that have helped shape this book or the thousands of people who have taken this challenge and changed their lives. And you certainly don't have to believe us just because we are saying these words. All you have to do is make a first-hand experience of life alcohol-free by taking this challenge. At this point you will be able to look at yourself in the mirror and know that you have experienced life once again, and done so alcohol-free. From this experience you can make the choice that's right for you.

> AF for 28 days – pros
> so far:
> - Weight loss
> - Best skin in years
> - Clearer eyes
> - Better rest
> - More centered in myself
> - Saved about £300
> As a result, this weekend I navigated some difficult personal circumstances in a calm, thoughtful and focused manner.
>
> **AMY**

— £15 a day
— £105 a week
— £420 **per month**
— £5040 **per year.**

Drinking from the ages of 18 to 68 would mean spending £252,000 on alcohol. Ridiculous. Let's throw in a bit of compound interest and it looks closer to £300,000, and let's not even consider the higher prices of wine or liquor! For couples saving for their first house, this is a sobering exercise. Both partners often consume a similar amount, which in the example above means a couple spending £600,000 or more on booze over their drinking lifetime.

MORE MONEY IN YOUR POCKET

Before embarking on our OneYearNoBeer challenge we had never questioned how much money we spent on alcohol. We guessed it was a lot, but we'd never dare do the maths for fear of discovering the truth – it was costing us a fortune.

Let's break it down. We know there are always hidden costs to drinking – cigarettes, taxis, takeaways – but for this example we will just stick to the cost of beer.

If we take a rough estimate of drinking three beers per day, with each (London) pint costing roughly £5, this equates to:

We fully appreciate the numbers above are very rough, and some drink a little less or a little more, but whatever way you look at it, the average drinking career costs a fortune.

Just imagine all the wonderful things you could do or buy with the money saved by not drinking? How great would it feel to have the extra cash to spend on those things you really enjoy? We all work so hard; why waste all this effort on a pastime that's holding you back?

Let's keep digging into this money pit: drinking alcohol can lead to poor health – both physical and mental – which has associated costs. Alcohol-related illness (aka hangovers) can prevent us exercising,

ANDY'S STORY

One of the hardest things about quitting alcohol is that you might end up different. I had used alcohol for years as liquid extroversion. Underneath the booze cloak I was really an introvert. Just imagine, for years I had convinced myself I was this flamboyant extrovert, but in truth this was a pretence fuelled by alcohol. I was always confused when I bumped into people the day after the night before, who expected more of the same, while all I wanted to do was go home, read, be with my family and learn stuff. In many ways I was living a lie. This made quitting alcohol even harder, because I knew this element of my persona might go.

I believe that of all the amazing advantages being alcohol-free brings, finding my authentic self is the greatest. I am so much happier, content and liberated now that I don't have to be that guy. I can now kick back and let others take on the mantle of extroversion. The pressure is off and I love it. For others like Ruari, you lift the booze cloak only to reveal exactly the same flamboyant, larger-than-life character. Ruari is no different with or without alcohol. He is quite happy to hold court and be the last man standing alcohol-free. Whether you are an introvert, extrovert, loud, quiet or shy, being true to yourself is a wonderful feeling.

which plays a part in heart disease, which in turn results in increased medical bills and insurance premiums. Taking too many sick days off work because of hangovers can cause you to miss out on deals and make you unreliable, affecting your opportunities for promotion. The price we really pay is almost impossible to calculate.

Whatever way you look at it, going alcohol-free provides a massive financial bonus. If you have something to save for or dreams that cost money, going alcohol-free is a wonderful way to free up extra cash.

DISCOVER YOUR AUTHENTIC SELF

There is something scary about taking a break from alcohol, something that we both agonised about. Like most people, we wanted to be accepted, liked and loved: going alcohol-free threatened our powerful craving for social acceptance and brought up some core fears. First, that we might be a different person without the alcohol and second, the fear of being labelled 'boring' or not the 'life and soul' any more.

We found ourselves asking the following questions:

— 'Will I be boring?'
— 'Will I be no fun without alcohol?'
— 'But what about Fun-Time-Four-Beers Andy?'

This was social conditioning at its most powerful: a sense that beneath the alcohol, our authentic selves might not be as much fun. But it was not until we had a decent break that we realized, for us, the opposite was true. One of the great achievements in life is to find your authentic self. There is something truly liberating about coming home to the real you. It's always there, it just gets lost at times, hijacked by alcohol and social conditioning.

It was not until we plucked up the courage to take on this challenge that we fully appreciated how good it felt to be ourselves, just as we are. It didn't matter if we were a little quieter – or a little louder in some cases. What mattered was that we were living lives that were authentic.

So don't be scared about losing face or being seen as 'different'. Take it from us – or our OYNBers – being your authentic self is one of life's great joys.

> *Anxiety has disappeared and in its place I have felt a peaceful openness. I still have stressful moments but I'm practising thinking about the stress before it consumes me. It's definitely work in progress as opposed to a demolition site. OYNB has helped enormously in getting me this far.*
>
> **THOMAS**

ANDY'S STORY

The morning-after anxiety I regularly experienced vanished. I count myself lucky that this anxiety was 100 per cent down to alcohol. Rather than creeping into my alcohol-free world, it simply disappeared. For me this was a massive win, as anyone who has suffered from anxiety and panic attacks will testify it's the most horrible feeling.

MIND FITNESS

Over the last few decades we have discovered just how important it is to exercise and eat well in order to maintain a healthy lifestyle. But we were both in danger of overlooking the most important part of the health puzzle: our mental health. Rather than an afterthought, building mental toughness should form the foundation of any healthy lifestyle and alcohol was playing havoc with ours. The nightly beer batterings often left us anxious, down and just not right. It was as if a cloud was constantly hanging over us.

Alcohol is a well-known depressant[66] and while it blocked out our emotions for a bit, they came back to haunt us the next day, which required blocking them out again – with alcohol. This vicious circle eroded our mental well-being, chipped away at our self-esteem and made us feel low. These marginal losses were starting to add up and anxiety crept into our everyday lives. To get over the anxiety we used alcohol, which in turn caused more anxiety.

For this reason we were both nervous about a life without alcohol. What if this anxiety raised its head and we had no way to deal with it? This is a major concern for many of our members and a massive reason why some people drink. They use alcohol as a form of self-medication, which then slowly becomes the problem. By removing alcohol from the equation we knew some of these issues might surface, but by meeting them with a clear head, we were confident that we could create a plan to deal with any problems that appeared.

The difference to our mental health was subtle yet powerful. We cannot state this enough: working on mental fitness is as, if not more, important than working on those abs. We both knew that if we could build a solid mental well-being base our physical health and diet would follow.

Next we experimented with techniques from the world of positive psychology, such as noting down three things we were grateful for each day. This was combined with a daily mindfulness (meditation) practice and physical exercise, which took our mental well-being to new highs.

Just like alcohol, there is a whole bucket of stigma attached to anything mental health. Although this is not the time and place to address these issues, we hope that by talking about this subject we can help reduce this stigma. Perhaps this is our next mission.

After 28 days I felt fairly invincible. I was amazed at how many 'firsts' I was experiencing and enjoying and, most importantly, learning from. It was so worth the down days of which there were quite a few ... but these just made me more determined. Signing up to the challenge gave me that accountability and a sense of belonging and that was priceless. I can't recommend it highly enough. Seriously, if you are thinking about it, either cutting down or cutting it out – how can you ever make a decision if you never give yourself the chance to experience a decent amount of time without alcohol? Now on day 95. Who knew?

SALLY

Once again, we genuinely believe if we had not taken a break from alcohol we would have missed the chance to work on our mind fitness – another massive alcohol-free advantage.

THE ONE THAT ENDS UP BEING FOUR

On reflection, we also realised that while drinking we often set out with the intention of having one drink but ended up having four. For some reason people feel the need to cover up this indiscretion. Out come little white lies: 'I only had one (four)', or 'I am just leaving now (two hours later).' At first these fibs went unnoticed, but once we no longer had to 'cover' for ourselves we both felt emotionally lighter. There was something freeing about not having to worry about tripping up over a previous half-truth. A healthy glow took over and we could look our partners in the eyes and know deep down that they knew the truth. When you first consider quitting alcohol, these types of benefits don't even compute because they are so subtle. Like all marginal gains, however, they add up to make a big difference.

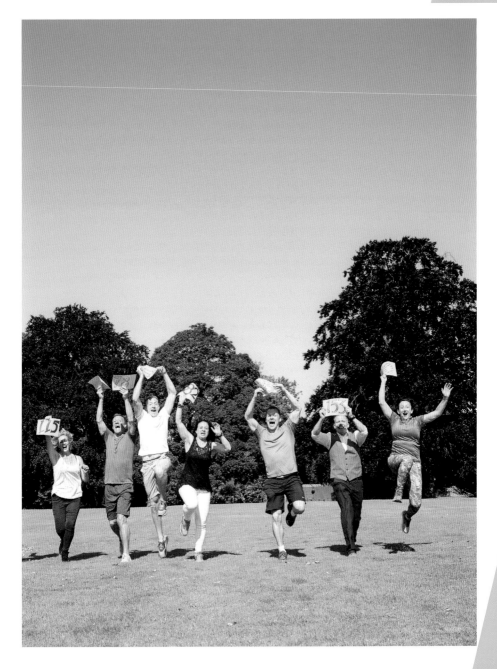

MORE HAPPINESS

The positive psychology movement has snowballed over the last decade, and so has the scientific understanding of happiness – or, as the positive psychologists like to call it, well-being. The brightest minds in the land are flocking to this new science to help unlock the big question in life: what actually makes us happy? And what does it mean to be happy?

Positive psychology aims to put those old wives' tales and life-coach wisdom to the test to discover what actually works and what doesn't. We are drawn to this field of study because it produces scientific evidence-based answers to many of our questions about well-being.

WELL-BEING

One of the first things we noticed about well-being is that everyone defines it differently. The clever bunch in white coats prefer the term well-being to happiness, which they break down into measurable components. From here science can work its brand of magic.

Positive psychology defines well-being through five elements: positive emotions, engagement, relationships, meaning and accomplishment (PERMA for short). Being alcohol-free supports and promotes every single one of these elements, producing a massive happiness gain.

> I smile so much more than I ever have done in my life. I look at the world through different eyes now. If you think about things in a positive way it helps you stay on target. I love chasing dreams, smashing goals and generally laughing. For the first time since I was 11 I don't need alcohol to do it. I can do it just being me, scary but true. I think I am a better, nicer, calmer and more in-control person.

AMIE

POSITIVE EMOTIONS

These are the classic feelings of happiness we experience when our football team wins or a child smiles at us.

As the mental fog of hangovers lifted and our inner worlds brightened, we got to experience laughter and to enjoy more activities that brought about feelings of positive emotions.

ENGAGEMENT

This is a state of flow athletes describe as being 'in the zone'. When we are engaged in something meaningful, time seems to stop and we are totally absorbed in the project.

As time formerly spent drinking came flooding back, we re-engaged in hobbies and interests that put us back in the zone.

RELATIONSHIPS

Meaningful, trusting relationships are essential to well-being.

One of the major advantages already discussed is how our relationships improved when we quit the drink. This helped us to experience more happiness.

MEANING

Believing in something bigger than oneself or supporting a cause can also pave the way to happiness[67].

Alcohol can provide 'plastic' meaning that melts the day after. Once alcohol-free, we had more time and space to look for authentic meaning in our lives.

ACCOMPLISHMENT

Pursuing achievement and mastery provides a sense of accomplishment that drives well-being.

As you can see, going alcohol-free enhances every single element of the well-being puzzle, freeing up energy to pursue dormant goals and dreams, creating another fantastic advantage.

While this list of advantages is far from exhaustive, it hopefully provides the sense that taking a break from alcohol provides myriad benefits which all feed each other to create a vibrant, healthy lifestyle.

I had a dinner party last night for my husband's birthday. We had our AF beers and the AF bubbles ready, but we spent most of the night just sipping on lime sodas. The rest of the crew who were drinking didn't even notice and it was a hilarious evening. And now we've just woken up, with clear minds, rested and ready for a day with the kids. In days past, we'd be in agony, exhausted, with hazy memories and probably with an alcohol-fuelled little tetchy argument about something stupid. Truly amazing. And so simple.

NICOLA

BREAK GLASS IN CASE OF EMERGENCY

Ok, so you're about to face a big social event. Don't panic! Take a deep breath and read the tips below. We start with the generic hacks for any event, then move into some specific tips for special occasions.

TIPS FOR ANY BIG SOCIAL OCCASION

KNOW EXACTLY WHAT YOU'RE GOING TO DRINK AND HAVE A BACK-UP PLAN (DAY 6)

This might sound over the top, but it's key to know exactly what you're going to drink. Phone the venue ahead of the event if you like, and have a back-up drink or two planned just in case your first choice in not available (Day 6).

USE VISUALISATION TO PREPARE LIKE A WORLD-CLASS ATHLETE (DAY 4)

Like an athlete uses visualisation to prepare for a competition, you should rehearse your alcohol-free evening in your mind.

READ YOUR REASONS WHY (DAY 1)

Refer to Day 1 when you made a list of all your reasons why you're here. Reminding yourself 'why' will keep you on track.

TALK TO THE RINGLEADERS (DAY 4)

If you are unsure about how your friends and colleagues will respond to this challenge, consider talking to the ringleaders first.

BRING A GOAL FRIEND (DAY 7)

It always helps to have some back-up, so why not bring a 'goal friend' along for some ready-made support?

USE THE EXCUSE (DAY 1)

Be ready to whip out your excuse – 'I am on a 28-day alcohol-free challenge and I'm loving it!'

REMEMBER: YOU DON'T HAVE TO DRINK IT JUST BECAUSE YOU OR SOMEONE ELSE BOUGHT IT (DAY 5)

ALWAYS HAVE AN ESCAPE ROUTE (DAY 5)

While alcohol-free parties can be off-the-scale fun, most people drinking alcohol are on a different planet come midnight. So always have an escape route to get you out early.

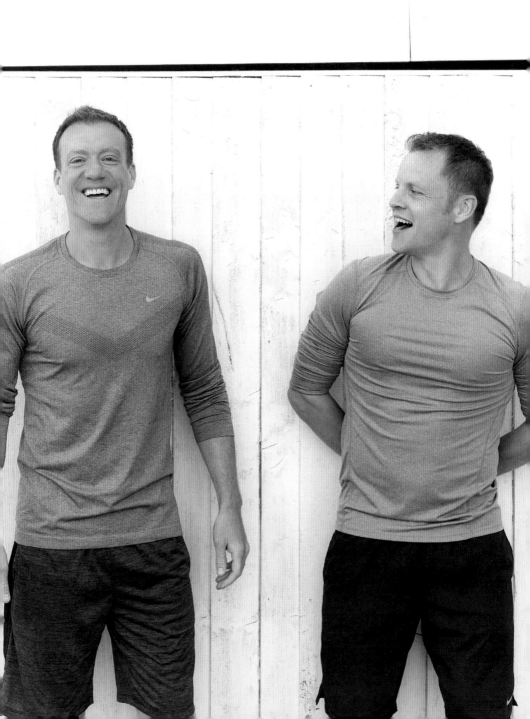

TURN THE NIGHT INTO A MICRO CHALLENGE (DAY 13)

The average night out lasts roughly five hours – that's all you have to survive. Why not make a game out of it and have fun? Score a point for every drunken snog you witness; two points for how many times your best mate says 'I love you!' and so on. The jackpot – dancing sober! Get creative and turn your event into five hours of fun.

TURN ON THE POWER OF LISTENING (DAY 4)

Aim to find out something new about a friend. Take time to listen deeply to what they have to say in a non-judgemental fashion. You might be surprised at what you discover.

ENJOY FEELING A LITTLE UNCOMFORTABLE BUT STILL YOUR TRUE SELF (DAY 8)

You might feel a little uncomfortable, but see this as a sign that you are being true to yourself and not bulldozing your emotions.

MINI FIST PUMP (DAY 4)

Surprisingly, many of the best challenge highlights happen after a big social challenge. So at the end of the night celebrate with a mini fist pump and perhaps treat yourself to something nice – you deserve it. The best treat of all, however, is waking up the following morning full of life and ready to take on the world!

THE AF HOLIDAY

Alcohol-free holidays rock – and the extra energy and vitality will make this your best one ever. As always, a bit of planning will make all the difference.

PHONE AHEAD

If you're staying in a hotel or resort, call ahead and check out all the alcohol-free options so you are prepared from day one.

EXERCISE

Use this as a chance to exercise daily. Perhaps treat yourself to a personal trainer or join in a yoga class.

MAKE A SUNRISE

A nice alcohol-free treat is to get up and on it just as the sun comes up somewhere beautiful. This is a great reminder of how life has changed for the better.

GET ACTIVE

Use your extra energy to try different types of activities. Push yourself to do something new. Perhaps go hiking or kayaking or try water polo. Enjoy feeling fresh and vibrant.

THE WEDDING

Weddings are one of those social occasions that many alcohol-free adventurers fear, but they are also the greatest social occasion to overcome. The discovery that you can truly enjoy an occasion such as this with a clear head is life changing, because in doing so you smash many of those long-held limiting beliefs around alcohol. You prove first hand that you can have a vibrant social life and still enjoy the big occasions without the booze.

THE CHAMPAGNE RECEPTION

Accommodating waiters are always ready to shove a glass of bubbles into your hand on arrival. Be ready - there is normally a soft-drink option, but if not smile and say, 'No thank you' and move on. Whatever happens, go out of your way to make sure you have a non-alcoholic drink to hold while mingling at this early stage. Having a drink in your hand will help you settle into the event.

THE DINNER

At many weddings the choice of drinks is limited, so you might have to freestyle. A great tip is to use a wine glass or champagne flute and fill it with sparking water. It will look like a real drink and will also feel somewhat special.

GET A ROOM

If you are staying over, try to book a room in the hotel where the wedding party is being held. This will provide a little oasis if you need to recharge your alcohol-free batteries and take a break.

CUT THE RUG

Weddings are the perfect place to experience the joys of sober dancing. No one cares what you look like or if you move like Jagger. Throw some shapes and see what happens. You might actually enjoy it!

THE STAG OR HEN

This really is the ultimate alcohol-free challenge, but if you can survive the stag or hen without booze, everything else will be a walk in the park.

Let's be honest, these events are pretty much about getting annihilated and making complete fools of yourselves. The trick to enjoying the stag or hen and still have everyone think you are a legend is to plan.

SHOTS

For every shot they take, have a shot of lime cordial. It's absolutely rank and you will get a massive high from all the sugar. Make a point of showing a disgusted face. If lime cordial isn't your thing, make it something equally horrid. The point is you are telling the crew that you are also suffering.

FLAGGING?

Have an energy drink. This is no time for weakness – and don't you dare be the first one back to the hotel. If anything, be the last.

ORCHESTRATE THEIR DRUNKENNESS

Be the first person to call out 'Shots!' Buy a bottle of something to shoot on the plane and be the naughty one passing it around – even bring the shot glasses or a hip flask. The gang will absolutely love you. They'll hate you in the morning, but who cares? It's a stag/hen! Your poor partner will just have to put up with your breath smelling of lime for the next six months.

From our experience, a number of things will happen during a stag/hen do:

— You will be cornered, quietly and individually, by everyone asking how you stopped, how you feel and why you are doing it. Everyone wants a break, but nobody wants to admit it.

— Be prepared to herd the crew, with people repeating themselves, getting lost and losing stuff. Sort them all out. They won't have a bad word to say about you once you've found their stuff, helped them home or listened to their life stories.

— You will wake up feeling amazing and proud that you didn't drink, but you might have a massive sugar crash. Bring enough paracetamol for everyone and be loved even more.

— The opposite sex will seek you out. There is something about being sober late on. You're standing upright, your face doesn't look like you're having a stroke and that seems to make you attractive to the opposite sex. Enjoy the attention, you legend!

Get the plan from the organiser early on and say that you can help make it run. Being the organiser or helping to organise the event will undoubtedly give you social kudos and you'll know when to back off because you'll be sober.

So, plan well, read up about some drinking games, take the (red) bull by the horns and be awesome!

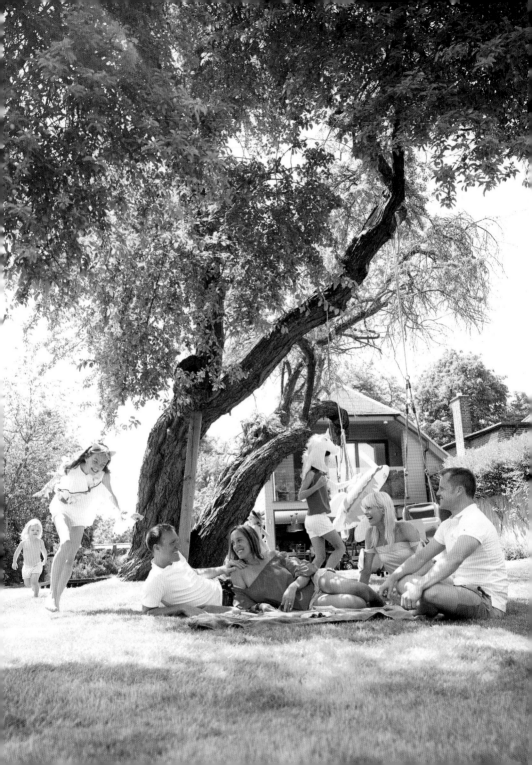

MOCKTAILS

When those special occasions come along and you don't want to miss out on the celebratory fun, why not make a little extra effort and whip up a few mocktails that will be the envy of their alcoholic rivals?

For these three mocktails we have enlisted the help of Seedlip, creator of the world's first non-alcoholic spirits. Seedlip is sugar-free, sweetener-free with no artificial flavours and zero calories – and we love it.

SEEDLIP GARDEN & TONIC

A brand new AF take on the classic G&T, with herby, grassy floral notes and refreshing zing. Makes one glass.

Ingredients
Handful of peas
50ml Seedlip Garden 108
125ml Indian tonic water

Method
Half fill a highball glass with ice cubes, interspersing the peas among the cubes. Pour over the Seedlip Garden 108, then top up with the tonic water. Serve at once.

SEEDLIP SPICE & TONIC

Aromatic, earthy and woody flavours abound with notes of cardamom and allspice as well as citrus top notes. Makes one glass.

Ingredients
50ml Seedlip Spice 94
125ml Indian tonic water
Grapefruit twist, to garnish

Method
Half fill a highball glass with ice cubes, pour over the Seedlip Spice, then top up with the tonic water. Garnish with the grapefruit twist and serve at once.

PENNSYLVANIA DUTCH

An elegant cocktail best served stirred, not shaken. Makes one glass.

Ingredients
60ml Seedlip Spice 94
20ml Raspberry Shrub★
Lemon twist, to garnish

Method
Stir the Seedlip and shrub over ice. Strain into a coupe glass and garnish with the lemon twist. Serve at once.

★Raspberry Shrub
Place 150g raspberries in a 500ml jar with 250ml apple cider vinegar and 225g white sugar. Muddle, leave overnight, then strain.

NOW FOR SOME SIMPLE, YET DELICIOUS SUGGESTIONS FROM OUR MEMBERS

It's so much fun playing around with flavours to make your own alcohol-free drinks. Here are just a few ideas from our members – but remember that if you combine delicious fresh flavours and balance out the sweet/ tangy elements, you'll usually end up with something great!

SPARKLING APPLE, ELDERFLOWER & MINT

This makes enough for around 8 servings, perfect for a garden party or barbecue.

Ingredients

75ml elderflower cordial
1 litre cloudy apple juice
Handful of chopped mint leaves
1 litre sparkling water

Method

Mix the elderflower and apple juice in a large jug. Throw in some mint leaves, stir. Half fill chilled glasses with the mixture. Top up with sparkling water.

TROPICAL PUNCH

A great drink to make on a hot day. Makes two glasses.

Ingredients

Two handfuls of favourite chopped fruits: strawberries, halved; kiwi fruit, peeled and chopped; pineapple, peeled, cored and chopped
150ml sparkling apple juice
150ml tropical fruit juice
150ml soda water

Method

Divide the chopped fruit between two highball glasses and add a couple of ice cubes to each. Add equal amounts of apple juice and tropical fruit juice and top up with soda water.

LIME AND MINT COOLER

If you're a fan of mojitos this should really hit the spot. Makes two glasses.

Ingredients

2 limes, cut into wedges
Handful fresh mint leaves, roughly chopped
2–4 tsp sugar, to taste
500ml soda water

Method

Divide the limes and mint between two sturdy glasses. Add 1 tsp sugar to each glass and muddle. Fill each glass with a crushed ice and top up with soda water. Stir and taste – add more sugar if needed.

RESOURCES

You can find links to all the resources below and much more on your dedicated '28-day challenge book' resources page at www.oneyearnobeer.com/book-resources.

And don't forget to check out our podcast: OneYearNoBeer – www.oneyearnobeer.com/podcasts/ Join authors Andy and Ruari on this fun ride into all things alcohol-free and healthy living.

MIND

Podcasts
Tim Ferris – tim.blog/podcast/
This podcast blows our mind on a regular basis. It's full of interesting guests from the worlds of mindfulness, business, sport and philosophy.
Lewis Howes – lewishowes.com/blog/
School of Greatness Podcast

Courses
Mindfulness – Search for an MBSR (Mindfulness Based Stress Relief) course near you. These courses are now widely available.

Apps
Headspace – This is our favourite meditation app and the perfect place to start.
Calm – Another wonderful meditation app and resource.

Books
Sane New World: Taming the Mind, Ruby Wax
Mindfulness: A Practical Guide to Finding Peace in a Frantic World, Mark Williams and Danny Penman
Full Catastrophe Living, Revised Edition: How to cope with stress, pain and illness using mindfulness meditation, Jon Kabat-Zinn
Search Inside Yourself: The Unexpected Path to Achieving Success, Happiness (and World Peace), Chade-Meng Tan
Awaken the Giant Within - Tony Robbins

Movements
www.alustforlife.com - A movement for all things wellbeing
www.actionforhappiness.org - A movement to make the world a happier place
www.mindbodygreen.com - For your daily wellness inspiration and news

EXERCISE

Podcast
The Rich Roll podcast – www.richroll.com/category/podcast/
Andy's favourite podcast, which dives deep into exercise, nutrition, spirituality and so much more.

Get fit
www.barrysbootcamp.com – the best workout in the world
www.virginactive.com – the world's leading health club

Apps
Strava – Connects millions of athletes via an easy-to-use app. It maps your runs and rides so that you can compare and compete against friends. We have a group called One Year No Beer – join up and race against Ruari and Andy.
Fitbit – This app tracks your steps and you can compete against OYNB members in the weekly Fitbit challenges if you join the OneYearNoBeer Fitbit group. (Requires a fitbit watch or accessory.)

Books
The First 20 Minutes: The Surprising Science of How We Can Exercise Better, Train Smarter and Live Longer, Gretchen Reynolds
Finding Ultra: Rejecting Middle Age, Becoming One of the World's Fittest Men, and Discovering Myself, Rich Roll
The 4-Hour Body: An Uncommon Guide to Rapid Fat-loss, Incredible Sex and Becoming Superhuman, Tim Ferriss

NUTRITION

Podcasts
No Meat Athlete – www.nomeatathlete.com/radio-archive/
This fun podcast will introduce you to many different nutritional ideas, although it's predominantly a plant-based, wholefoods approach.
The Model Health Show – theshawnstevensonmodel.com/podcasts/

Courses
Joe Wicks, The Body Coach – www.thebodycoach.com
The 90-day SSS online course is one of the world's leading tailored fat-loss plans.
Amanda Hamilton – amandahamilton.com
Nutritional retreats and clinic.

Books
Lean in 15 – The Shift Plan: 15 Minute Meals and Workouts to Keep You Lean and Healthy, Joe Wicks
How Not To Die: Discover the foods scientifically proven to prevent and reverse disease, Dr Michael Greger with Gene Stone
The Paleo Solution: The Original Human Diet, Robb Wolf
The World of the Happy Pear, Stephen & David Flynn
I Quit Sugar: Your Complete 8-Week Detox Program and Cookbook, Sarah Wilson
Deliciously Ella Every Day: Simple recipes and fantastic food for a healthy way of life, Ella Mills
Nourish and Glow: The 10 Day Plan, Amelia Freer

DO

Groups

Parkrun – www.parkrun.com
This fantastic FREE timed 5k run takes place all over the world at 9 a.m. every saturday morning.
Nuclear races – nuclear-races.co.uk/
Tough, gritty award winning fun obstacle races.
Meetup – www.meetup.com/
Think of a hobby you love and there will be a meetup somewhere near you. This is a wonderful way to meet new people.
Open university – www.open.ac.uk
Perhaps this challenge will unlock the time and energy to study?
toughmudder.co.uk – create the ultimate muddy challenge.
Spartanrace.uk – tough races with plenty of mud and obstacles.
www.britishcycling.org.uk – get into cycling.

HABITS AND WILLPOWER

Books

The Power of Habit: Why We Do What We Do,
and How to Change, Charles Duhigg
The Willpower Instinct, Kelly Mcgonigal

Habit change system

Pavlock - www.pavlock.com

ALCOHOL FREE

Social

morninggloryville.com – the original morning rave.
daybreaker.com – the morning party that starts your day with energy & intention.
redemptionbar.co.uk – healthy food and delicious AF drinks.

Festivals

The OYNB Spitalfields Market: Happy AF Festival – www.oneyearnobeer.com/festival
The world's largest AF festival

Movements

hellosundaymorning.org - change your drinking habits.
Club Soda - joinclubsoda.co.uk.
The Mindful Drinking Movement
soberistas.com – love life in control.
This Naked Mind – thisnakedmind.com

GO ALCOHOL FREE FOR CHARITY

Alcohol Concern – alcoholconcern.org.uk.
  Promoting health, improving lives and creators of the Dry January campaign
Help for Heroes – helpforheroes.org.uk.
  Supporting the injured armed forces.
Cancer Research – cancerresearchuk.org.
  Bringing forward the day when all cancers are cured.
Charity Water – charitywater.org.
  Brings clean, safe drinking water to people in need.
Georgia's Teenage Cancer Appeal – gtca-appeal.org.
Wipe away Those Tears – wipeawaythosetears.org
  Bringing a sparkle into the lives of terminally or seriously ill children.
Drinkaware – drinkaware.co.uk.
  Working to reduce alcohol related misuse and harm in the uk.
Go sober for October – www.gosober.org.uk.
  Raise money for Macmillan cancer nurses.
Marie Curie – mariecurie.org.uk.
  Helping those with terminal illness.
British Heart Foundation – bhf.org.uk.
Alzheimers Society – alzheimers.org.uk.

 Find out more about Dry January and download their free app, Dry January & Beyond, at www.dryjanuary.org.uk

ENDNOTES

[1] www.independent.co.uk/life-style/food-and-drink/features/how-britain-scaled-peak-booze-2004-marked-the-high-water-mark-in-our-relationship-with-alcohol-a6721566.html

[2] www.huffingtonpost.com/russell-rosenberg-phd/alcohol-sleep_b_902578.html

[3] www.health.harvard.edu/heart-health/5-ways-to-de-stress-and-help-your-heart

[4] www.psychologytoday.com/blog/the-real-story-risk/201211/the-thing-we-fear-more-death

[5] J. Poilvy, C.P. Herman and R. Deo, 'Getting a Bigger Slice of the Pie: Effects on Eating and Emotion in Restraining and Unrestrained Eaters', *Appetite* 55 (2010): 426–30

[6] Steve Peters, *The Chimp Paradox: The Mind Management Programme to Help You Achieve Success, Confidence and Happiness* (London, Vermilion, 2012)

[7] www.nhs.uk/Livewell/fitness/Pages/whybeactive.aspx

[8] www.brainyquote.com/quotes/quotes/m/marktwain122378.html

[9] A. Baikie, K. Wihelm. 'Emotional and Physical Health Benefits of Expressive Writing', *Advances in Psychiatric Treatment* (2005), vol. 11: 338–346

[10] http://news.cornell.edu/stories/2006/02/candy-desk-candy-mouth-study-finds

[11] Understanding the relationship between food environments, deprivation and childhood overweight and obesity: Evidence from a cross sectional England-wide study. *Health & Place* (2014), vol. 27: 68-76

[12] Charles Duhigg, *The Power of Habit: Why We Do What We Do and How to Change* (London, Random House, 2012)

[13] ibid.

[14] Gretchen Reynolds, *The First 20 Minutes: The Surprising Science of How We Can Exercise Better, Train Smarter and Live Longer* (London, Penguin, 2012)

[15] ibid.

[16] Shawn Stevenson, *Sleep Smarter: 21 Essential Strategies to Sleep Your Way to a Better Body, Better Health, and Bigger Success* (New York, Rodale, 2016)

[17] www.thoughtco.com/using-visualization-to-succeed-in-basketball-326408#step3

[18] www.news.appstate.edu/2011/06/13/early-morning-exercise/

[19] Robert Goldman and Stephen Papson, *Nike Culture: The Sign of the Swoosh* (Thousand Oaks, California, Sage Publications, 1999)

[20] M.R. Leary, C.E Tate, C.E. Adams, A.B. Allen and J. Hancock, 'Self-compassion and Reactions to Unpleasant Self-Relevant Events: The Implications of Treating Oneself Kindly', *Journal of Personality and Social Psychology* 92 (2007): 887–904

[21] www.drinkaware.co.uk/research/data/consumption-uk/

[22] www.quotes.net/citizen-quote/197503

[23] Kelly McGonigal, *Maximum Willpower: How to Master the New Science of Self-Control* (London, Penguin, 2012)

[24] www.brainyquote.com/quotes/quotes/u/usainbolt447704.html

[25] www.bbc.co.uk/sport/olympics/19174302

[26] Kelly McGonigal, *Maximum Willpower: How to Master the New Science of Self-Control* (London, Penguin, 2012)

[27] Richard Layard, *Happiness: Lessons from a New Science* (New York, Penguin Press, 2005)

[28] Tim Ferris, *The 4-Hour Body: An Uncommon Guide to Rapid Fat-loss, Incredible Sex and Becoming Superhuman* (London, Vermilion, 2011)

[29] www.nhs.uk/Livewell/Goodfood/Pages/the-eatwell-guide.aspx, accessed 19 May 2017

[30] www.azquotes.com/author/22527-Jason_Vale

[31] www.telegraph.co.uk/news/2016/12/28/8-10-middle-aged-adults-dangerously-unhealthy-says-government/

[32] Kelly McGonigal, *Maximum Willpower: How to Master the New Science of Self-Control* (London, Penguin, 2012)

[33] ibid.

[34] Steve Peters, *The Chimp Paradox: The Mind Management Programme to Help You Achieve Success, Confidence and Happiness* (London, Vermilion, 2012)

[35] Charles Duhigg, *The Power of Habit: Why We Do What We Do and How to Change* (London, Random House, 2012)

[36] M.E.P. Seligman, *Flourish* (New York, Free Press, 2011)

[37] N.A. Christakis, 'Social Networks and Collateral Health Effects', *BMJ* (2004), 329:184–5.

[38] Daniel Kahneman, *Thinking, Fast and Slow* (London, Penguin, 2012)

[39] Anthony Robbins, *Awaken the Giant Within: How to Take Immediate Control of Your Mental, Emotional, Physical and Financial Life* (London, Simon & Schuster, 2001)

[40] www.drinkaware.co.uk/alcohol-facts/health-effects-of-alcohol/mental-health/alcohol-and-mental-health/

[41] www.health.harvard.edu/heart-health/5-ways-to-de-stress-and-help-your-heart

[42] www.goodreads.com/quotes/978-whether-you-think-you-can-or-you-think-you-can-t--you-re

[43] Charles Duhigg, *The Power of Habit: Why We Do What We Do and How to Change* (London, Random House, 2012)

[44] Andy Puddicombe, *Get Some Headspace: 10 Minutes Can Make All the Difference* (London, Hodder, 2012)

45 P. Grossman, L. Niemann, S. Schmidt and H. Walach, 'Mindfulness-based Stress Reduction and Health 'Benefits: A Meta-analysis', *Journal of Psychosomatic Research*, (2004) 57: 35–43.

46 Charles Duhigg, *The Power of Habit: Why We Do What We Do and How to Change* (London, Random House, 2012)

47 www.brainyquote.com/quotes/authors/m/mike_tyson.html

48 M.E.P. Seligman, *Flourish* (New York, Free Press, 2011)

49 www.goodreads.com/quotes/6513400-it-is-not-that-we-have-a-short-time-to

50 Mark Williams and Danny Penman, *Mindfulness: A Practical Guide to Finding Peace in a Frantic World* (London, Piatkus, 2011)

51 en.wikiquote.org/wiki/Epictetus

52 Speech at Harrow School, 29 October 1941

53 Kelly McGonigal, *Maximum Willpower: How to Master the New Science of Self-Control* (London, Penguin, 2012)

54 www.psychologytoday.com/blog/the-science-willpower/201111/how-mindfulness-makes-the-brain-immune-temptation

55 Matthew Syed, *Black Box Thinking: Marginal Gains and the Secrets of High Performance* (London, John Murray, 2016)

56 Susan Cain, *Quiet: The Power of Introverts in a World That Can't Stop Talking* (London, Penguin, 2013)

57 Kelly McGonigal, *Maximum Willpower: How to Master the New Science of Self-Control* (London, Penguin, 2012).

58 www.brainyquote.com/quotes/quotes/l/laotzu118352.html

59 M.E.P. Seligman, *Flourish* (New York, Free Press, 2011)

60 Ryan Holiday, *Ego is the Enemy: The Fight to Master Our Greatest Opponent* (London, Profile Books, 2016)

61 N.A. Christakis, 'Social Networks and Collateral Health Effects', *BMJ* (2004), 329:184–5.

62 Elaine Fox, *Rainy Brain Sunny Brain: The New Science Of Optimism and Pessimism* (London, Arrow Books, 2012)

63 www.shinrin-yoku.org/shinrin-yoku.html

64 www.brainyquote.com/quotes/quotes/h/henrydavid104516.html

65 Gretchen Rubin, *Better Than Before: Mastering the Habits of Our Everyday Lives* (London, Two Roads, 2015)

66 www.drinkaware.co.uk/alcohol-facts/health-effects-of-alcohol/mental-health/alcohol-and-mental-health/

67 M.E.P Seligman, *Authentic Happiness: Using the New Positive Psychology to Realize Your Potential for Lasting Fulfillment* (New York, Free Press, 2002)

INDEX

ACKNOWLEDGEMENTS

From the authors

Firstly we would like to thank Jane Graham-Maw our wonderful book agent who has shared our AF mission from the outset.

We would like to thank our fantastic publisher Bluebird for fully aligning with our goal to make this a fun, upbeat, bright and inspirational book. We knew Bluebird were the ones for us when Carole Tonkinson and Jodie Mullish listened to our story as if it was the first they had ever heard. Thank you to our wonderful editor Katy Denny who has taken our rough diamond and given it a good old polish and to Ruth Jenkinson for the great photos. Also thank you to our nutritionists Jolene Park and Angela Dowden for expert guidance.

A massive thank you to those thought leaders and mentors that have moulded the ideas and techniques contained within this book – Anthony Robbins, Dan Meredith, Colm Carroll, Gary Vaynerchuk, Gretchen Rubin, Arianna Huffington, Tony Stubblebine, Johann Hari, Stanton Peele, Tara Brach, Shawn Achor, Carol Dweck, Brené Brown, Daniel Kahneman, and Malcolm Gladwell.

The PFA (Professional Footballers Association) John Hudson for sharing the vision that this AF challenge could improve the health of supporters all over the world over. Also thank you to Crawfurd Hill for his boundless enthusiasm for this project and his early input.

Special thank you to Rich Roll for being our mentor and hero. Also Stephen Flynn and David Flynn aka The Happy Pear for showing the world that you can have the most fun without drinking. Thank you to Ollie Ollerton who demonstrates on a daily basis that real men don't have to drink. Also a special mention to Pat Divilly, Ireland's no. 1 performance coach, for being such a wonderful support in everything we do.

To those mega cool celebrities who inspired us to write the book by showing that you can be a superstar, create wonderful things and not drink – thank you.

Tom Hardy, Freddie Flintoff, Russell Brand, Rich Roll, Bear Grylls, Peter Kay, Bradley Cooper, Tim McGraw, Colin Farrell, Robert Downey Jr, Ben Affleck, John Travolta, Daniel Radcliffe, Lenny McAuliffe, Bruce Willis, Chris Martin, Eric Clapton, David Walliams, Calvin Harris, Ewan McGregor, Simon Pegg, Paul Stenton, Lisa Jordan, Michelle Bridges and Ashling Keenan.

Thank you to Joe Kelly and Javier Loya of OTC Global Holdings for having the foresight to be the first to help us promote this movement and for their ongoing assistance. Also we must mention Richard Taggart, Niki Balac and Jamie Spicer of Aalpha Energy for the daily support they offer to Andy.

We must thank David Hufton, Simon Andrews, Iain Gilligan, Helen Post and all of the PVM team, especially Callum, Alex and Phil on the Jet desk. All of whom not only put up with Ruari, but go out of their way to support the project.

Finally a massive eternal thanks to all our ambassadors, the moderators and those who have helped the OYNB community become what it is today. It's your voice that has made OYNB the most special place on the internet, with your guidance and constant watching and supporting. Thanks especially to Christine Penrose, Anna Stokes, Michael Gonsalves, Andrea Adnan, Stephanie Chivers, Karl Elliott, Elizabeth Canavan, Helen Randle, Felicia MacIntyre, Andy Leighton, Mark Rees, Kate Goodman, Charlotte Sutherland, Liz Ottoson, Jarlath Galantly, Amie Symonds, Denis Pickering, Joanne Gibson, Alan Desmond, Nick Read and Lisa Knight.

From the publisher

The team at Bluebird would like to give huge thanks to Stoke Place for welcoming us to their grounds and hotel to take photos; the OYNB members who gave up a Saturday morning to come along for some group shots; Ruari and Jen for letting us take photos in their lovely home; Jen, Robin, Tillie, Tara, Molly and Ruby for being such great models.